# TO YOUR HEALTH

GEORGE AYOUB, PhD

## DEDICATION

In loving memory of my parents, who nurtured me onto the path of thinking creatively and making the world a better place. Thank you for your hard work, inspiration and love. And for my child, who shows me every day how beautiful life is. I love you.

# CONTENTS

# Introduction

This book explains how your body works to help you decide what you can do to improve the health of you and your family. Throughout this book, I use knowledge gained in a career as an educator and scientist. I've taught 10,000 university students in biology and psychology and neuroscience, and have been doing biomedical research for more than thirty years. I've taught a wide range of courses, including high school and college, graduate and medical school, and have trained physicians, health professionals, scientists, as well as artists, writers, and community workers. This range of teaching has helped me explain complex medical topics clearly.

From teaching, I learned that everyone likes to know about their health, and that it is easiest to learn when someone uses normal language and examples that are to the point.

This book has chapters by topic, and you can read them in any order you wish. It is written so you can pick it up and just read the subject you need at the moment. I introduce some medical terms with each subject and use them in the descriptions and explanations. This is intentional. It is common to be in a medical setting with someone close to you who is ill, and you need to be the person who talks with the medical staff. Knowing some of the medical words helps you understand things. I try to include the most common medical words for you to understand what is being said and have the courage to speak. Remember in those moments: you are the voice for your loved one.

Our bodies are impressive. Starting from a single cell the size of a pencil dot, this develops into organs and tissues that take in nutrients and energy, filter air and liquids, build materials, process information, move about, sense the world in many ways, communicate, fight infection, and create things that have never existed. Each of these actions involves many body parts working together, keeping us in balance. I find it fascinating and have marveled at it all, much as the Psalmist, who said, "I am fearfully and wonderfully made" (Psalm 139).

Just over a century ago, the vast majority of us died of infectious disease. We rarely lived long enough to get sick from chronic (i.e., long-term) diseases. It is estimated that 90 percent of the population died of infectious diseases in the eighteenth and nineteenth centuries, with only 10 percent dying of chronic disease like heart disease or cancer. Today these numbers are reversed in most of the developed world And with immunizations we have little fear of infectious disease; you are more likely to be hit with a chronic disease.

How did this come about? Mostly by two great successes in medical history. The first is access to clean water, which has substantially reduced the spread of disease because we are able to wash ourselves and keep germs from entering our bodies. The second is immunizations, antibiotics and other modern medicines that have controlled infectious diseases. So we live in a wondrous time for health. We have all the tools to live a productive and healthy life. The bigger challenges now are to learn to use this medical knowledge and apply what we know about chronic diseases to make life better for us and our families.

Now that most of us live long enough to get a chronic disease, we also have a risk of becoming unable to answer what we want done if we get very sick. Doctors cannot make decisions about our health for us, so to protect your rights, it is wise to complete an Advance Directive, also called an Advance Health Care Directive. Forms to make a Directive are available through doctor's offices and clinics. What the Directive does is indicate in general what you want done if you cannot respond to the doctor, and who you want to make any decisions for you. The decision-maker is usually someone close to you, who knows what you want, and the Directive lets the medical team know that this person can speak for you when you are unable to do so.

What we know about health is not secret. Many studies are published. But this information is often overlooked because we are so busy that each of us cannot look up every study to know what to do in our life. The things that do improve our health, like what we eat and our daily activity, are inexpensive. They are available for everyone. Often, because this involves simpler things, it gets overlooked. But ignoring these simple things means we need expensive medicines to fight off a disease when we could prevent many chronic diseases with our simple actions and common foods.

Let's see how to do it.

*Overview*

This book goes through the systems of our body and explains the major principles behind having a healthy life. There are three key categories of how we can improve our health: Foods, Activities, Environment. Each of these are summarized here.

Foods: having a diet that is mostly vegetables, fruits and fish, using monounsaturated fats; reducing or eliminating red meat, burnt foods and saturated fats.

Activities: keeping physically active throughout life by moving your body every day for 30-60 minutes. When younger, this activity is typically more strenuous, and less so as we age.

Environment: getting regular medical checkups, being aware of areas that affect you the most (perhaps due to family history), not smoking (cigarettes, vaping or other form), minimizing exposure to pesticides and toxins, reducing stress and getting good sleep.

# From Atoms to Cells and Organs

Everything we see, everywhere, is made of atoms. Atoms are the simplest unit of all matter. Every solid, liquid or gas is made of atoms. And atoms have a structure to them that creates their properties. There are just over 100 different types of atoms, which are called the elements, and these different atoms makes up everything we see.

We understand atoms today based on their structure that makes them: the nucleus made of protons and neutrons and electrons that orbit around the nucleus. These three kinds of particles are key to the structure and function of the different types of atoms. In the late 1800s, before anyone knew about these atomic particles, scientists were able to figure out the properties of the different elements. In fact, it was from the observations about the properties of different types of atoms that Mendeleev made the first periodic table of the elements. His chart categorized all the elements known at the time, and it also predicted elements not yet undiscovered. What Mendeleev came up with was that the number of protons and electrons in an atom is what controlled how that atom would function. He arranged all the elements into rows and columns based on these interactions. It turned out the rows and columns he came up with were directly due to the numbers of protons and electrons the atom had.

An element is something made of one type of atom. For example, a block of carbon or a diamond is made only of carbon atoms. There are over 100 elements, with each named by the number of protons it has. If it has one proton, it is the first element, if 8 protons it is the eighth element.

Protons and electrons are particles that make up atoms. Protons have a positive charge, electrons have a negative charge. Atoms also have neutrons, which have no charge. Protons and neutrons have about the same mass, and their mass is referred to as an atomic unit. Electrons are much lighter, about a thousandth the mass of a proton or neutron.

The heavier protons and neutrons clump together to form the nucleus of the atom, and the electrons circle around the nucleus. The nucleus makes up most of the mass of the atom, but the electrons are important in making controlling how atoms work. Each element is named by how many protons it has, with hydrogen, the first element, having one proton, and helium, the second element, having two. Atoms generally have as many electrons circling the nucleus as the number of protons in the nucleus.

All the electrons of atoms are in orbit around the nucleus in what are called orbitals, with each orbital further from the nucleus. So, the first orbital is closest, the second is next, and so on. In this way, atoms with one or two electrons have these electrons in the first orbital, but once the atom has more than two electrons, it needs to have electrons in the second orbital, which is further from the nucleus. This second orbital can hold up to eight electrons, and when the atom has more than ten electrons in total (2 in first, 8 in second orbitals), electrons begin to fill the third orbital (which has room for 8 more electrons. The fourth and fifth orbitals can hold up to 18 electrons each, and the sixth and seventh orbitals can have up to 32 electrons in each.

## Periodic Table of the Elements

The rows of the periodic table indicate the number of electron orbitals used by a particular element. Hydrogen and helium are on the first row, and these are the only two elements using only one orbital. The further out from the nucleus the orbital is, the more energy it takes to have the electron there. This means that electrons will always go to the lowest orbital available, and if an electron moves to a higher orbital (for example, when the atom is hit with a pulse of electricity), the electron will quickly return to its lower orbital. When it returns, it gives off energy, and this energy can be seen by us as light. In fact, this is how fluorescent lights work. The phosphors inside the bulb are hit with a high energy electrical pulse, which knocks some electrons into higher orbitals. These electrons immediately return to their normal orbital and give off energy, which we see as light.

The rows of the table indicate the number of electron orbitals, with the top row indicating elements with one orbital, the second row has two orbitals, and so on. The columns, from left to right, indicate how many electrons are in the outermost orbital for the element. Atoms in the column on the right have a full set of electrons in their orbitals. These atoms are the most stable of all the elements, and will not interact with other atoms. Because they do not interact with the other elements, these elements are known as the noble elements, as they share a trait of the old kings and queens (nobility) in that they do not interact with the commoners.

In contrast, elements in the left-most column have only one electron in their outer orbital. These elements will be more stable if they can share that electron, and so these elements are very reactive, sharing that electron with another element. Sodium and hydrogen are in this left column, and these elements will violently react with anything that will take that extra electron.

On the right side of the chart, next to the noble elements, is a column (one line in from the right) where each element is just one electron shy of having a full outer orbital. These elements are intensely reactive, and will try to grab an electron from something else in order to fill this orbital. Chlorine and fluorine are in this second from the right column, and these aggressively strip an electron from another element to help stabilize them. This is why bleach uses chlorine, as it will react quickly, and we then use this bleach to remove color from things.

A common substance formed from these volatile elements is salt, which is a combination of sodium and chlorine (NaCl). While salt is comprised of two of the most highly reactive elements, it is completely calm since the excess electron from the sodium (Na) is shared with chlorine (Cl) to make the pair more stable together than separate.

*Molecules*

Electron sharing is how molecules are formed. Molecules are compounds made of more than one atom. The atoms bind together by sharing electrons in what is called a covalent bond. By sharing electrons, the two atoms are each more stable in combination, since they each have an outer electron orbital this is full (the most stable condition). By sharing electrons, the atoms are more stable as a molecule than when they are apart. Because the bond creates stability, there is a lot of energy in a covalent bond.

All atoms except the noble elements can form one or more covalent bonds. The number of bonds each atom can have is determined by how many electrons are needed to have a full outer orbital. Sodium and hydrogen can form one covalent bond, while oxygen can form two and carbon can form four. Carbon is the lightest element that can form four bonds. Carbon is the atom that is in all molecules that make up life.

Molecules that are made up of a chain of carbon atoms attached to each other are called organic molecules, which means they are molecules that form the living things. Depending on what other atoms are attached to these carbons, these organic molecules will be in one of the four categories named next.

If the carbon atoms are in a line, each connected to another carbon and having hydrogen atoms in the other carbon bonds, we call this molecule a hydrocarbon (named for its parts: hydrogen and carbon). Hydrocarbons are oils, and these form the edges of every cell in our bodies. Hydrocarbons, also called as lipids or fats when they are in our body, are used to store energy for our bodies in the form of fat, or energy that we use for commercial fuel in the form of petroleum or other oils. The reason we use hydrocarbons for carrying energy is that hydrocarbons have a lot of bonds that hold energy (the carbon to carbon bonds), and this energy can be given off for other uses by enzymes in the body or by burning fuel in a heater or an engine. Hydrocarbons are so energy intensive that they hold twice the energy as the next energy molecule used in our bodies.

When the each of the carbons in a molecule are connected to water, with hydrogen on one side and oxygen plus hydrogen on the other, this has the effect of adding one water for each carbon, water is made of two hydrogens and one oxygen. We call this molecule a carbohydrate, because the carbon is hydrated (it has water added). Carbohydrates are the most common form of energy that we consume and use in our body. In fact, our blood always has the carbohydrate glucose in it, because glucose is used by all our cells to make energy inside the cell. While carbohydrate has half the energy of fat, the energy is quickly converted to a form that we can use in our cells, so these nutrients provide energy for our regular activities.

So, these two large molecules, hydrocarbons and carbohydrates, are made from a chain of carbon that has hydrogen or water on each carbon. And these are two of the four macromolecules (large molecules) that make up our cells. The other two are proteins and DNA. Proteins are made of carbon, hydrogen, oxygen and nitrogen, while nucleic acids are made of the same four as proteins with phosphorus. Proteins are molecules in our cells that do work, moving, making new molecules or transmitting signals. All the enzymes in our cells are made of proteins, so proteins are how we make all the molecules in our cells. Nucleic acids are molecules that carry the information about how to make proteins. These nucleic acids are in the nucleus of the cell in a molecule called DNA (deoxyribonucleic acid), and carried to other areas of the cell where the proteins are actually made by a similar molecule called RNA (ribonucleic acid).

One more thing about hydrocarbons. You may have heard of saturated and unsaturated fats. Saturated means that every carbon bond that can be filled with a hydrogen is, while unsaturated means that some carbon bonds do not have a hydrogen (when this is the case, the carbons form an extra bond with each other). Oils can be mono-unsaturated (one unsaturated bond) or polyunsaturated (many of these bonds). The cooking oils that we currently think are healthier for us are not saturated. Animal fats are made of saturated fats. When a fat molecule is saturated, the individual hydrocarbons form a straight line, while if there is an unsaturated area, that part of the molecule has a bend in it. Because these straight line (saturated) hydrocarbons can pack more tightly, saturated fats are usually solid at room temperature, while unsaturated fats are liquid because they pack more loosely.

Another substance related to hydrocarbons is alcohol. Alcohol is almost a hydrocarbon, but it has one oxygen in it. This means that alcohols are also high energy molecules. They can be burned and give off a lot of energy, which is why motors can run on alcohol or on hydrocarbon fuel. But this high energy content also comes at a price for us. For the type of alcohol that we can drink (ethanol) gives us a lot of extra high energy carbon bonds, so by drinking alcohol we can quickly add to our daily calories without realizing how much we have added. This is why individuals who drink more alcohol are at risk to add extra fat on their body, as we see when someone has a "beer belly."

### Cells and Organelles

All cells are made from these four macromolecules, and also have vitamins, minerals and water. The membrane of each cell is made of lipids, which keeps the inside and outside of the cell separate. Since lipids (like all hydrocarbons) do not mix with water, they are hydrophobic (meaning they fear water, or do not mix with water). Membrane lipids have phosphates on their ends (next to the inside of the cell and next to the outside of the cell), and these phosphates do mix with water, meaning they are hydrophilic (water loving). Since we are primarily water based (our bodies are about 70% water), the phospholipid forms a waterproof barrier around each cell to keep the internal contents and the external contents from mixing. This means that cells have different conditions inside and outside, but it also means that cells need transport things across their membrane when needed.

In addition to the nucleus, cells have other compartments that have particular functions. Most of these structures are organelles, which are compartments in a cell that have one specific function. Mitochondria are one such organelle. The inside of the mitochondria work to convert glucose (the type of carbohydrate that circulates in the blood to provide energy to the cell) into the form of energy used by cells. Mitochondria take in glucose and oxygen and break the covalent bonds in glucose to free up its energy. The energy in glucose is converted inside the mitochondria to a type of energy called ATP (adenosine triphosphate). ATP is used inside cell, providing the energy all cells use, whether it's for moving our muscles, moving components around inside cells, assembling proteins, or something else.

### Tissues and Organs

Cells are grouped together in our body to make tissues. A tissue is a group of cells that work together for the same purpose. There are just four types of tissues: muscle, which moves us, epithelial, which makes the linings of all our organs and skin, connective, which provides support and protection through the body and is the most common type of tissue, and nervous, which conveys and processes information.

Some tissues are grouped together to make organs, like the heart, which has all four types of tissues working together to move blood. Some large functions are handled by organ systems, which are made of multiple organs and tissues. An example of an organ system is the digestive system, which has multiple organs working together to digest and store nutrients from the foods we eat.

# Beginnings

Each of us starts as a single cell. The first cell for any person is made by the combination of an egg and a sperm, which unite to make the first cell from which all the cells in our body arise. A human egg (called an oocyte) is the largest of human cells because it has not only the genetic code in the form of chromosomes made of DNA, but also it has all the cellular components and stored energy for this cell to reproduce many thousands of times before it can take begins to take in new energy sources. This means that the cytoplasm of the egg cell, which contains the energy making parts of our cells, must have enough nutrients to not only live but to expand its role tremendously. The information for what these dividing cells need to do is all coded in our DNA. Since we receive approximately half our DNA from each parent, and this DNA is arrayed in tens of thousands of genes (the units of chromosomes that define the code for each protein), that means all the things that define us are inherited from our biological parents genes.

In receiving half our genes from each parent, we collect two copies of most genes (one from each biological parent). Because there are small variations in the DNA codes for many genes, this means the two copies vary from each other slightly. This small variation is what gives rise to the visible differences between each of us, but also some more subtle differences in the proteins we produce. While each of the genes still has the code for the same overall protein, the small variations result in small differences in function. In this way, one adult may be able to digest milk, for example and another one not, or someone may be able to process alcohol or various foods more efficiently than another. We will discuss this variation in the chapter on digestion. It is this small variation within the genes that also creates rare genetic conditions that are handed down in families. For example, a person that inherits the S variant of hemoglobin (this is the molecule that carries oxygen in our blood) may have sickle cell anemia. We will discuss this in the cardiovascular chapter.

As you will see, our genes have a lot of information that determines not only how we grow and what we look like, but can influence the diseases we are susceptible to. Additionally, there are some variations in the cytoplasm of our cells between individuals, and since the cytoplasm is inherited only from the maternal side, it is a little easier to track these variations.

Because the cytoplasm comes only from the maternal egg cell, then all the cytoplasm and organelles are handed down to each person from the mother alone. Indeed, it is because our cytoplasm is maternally inherited that scientists can look at the genetic DNA that is passed along in the energy making organelles called the mitochondria. This bit of DNA can only be inherited from your biological mother, and due to this fact scientists have been able to extrapolate by the variations in this DNA to when the first human mother was around (this is calculated based on how many years it takes for random mutations to occur, and how many mutations we find in mitochondrial DNA). This person is referred to as Mitochondrial Eve.

In a similar fashion, only males have a Y chromosome, and so this one chromosome can only come from a male. By evaluating the mutations in the Y chromosomes seen today, one can estimate when the first human male was around. The estimates place both the Mitochondrial Eve and the Y Chromosome Adam as existing roughly the same time, about 100,000 to 200,000 years ago.

## Development

Once an egg is fertilized, the DNA in the sperm nucleus joins the egg nucleus to combine with the DNA there. Egg and sperm cells are unique in having only half the number of chromosomes (one of each pair instead of two), so once the two nuclei unite, the fertilized egg has a full set of DNA. This genetic information determines the production of all proteins in the cell. Since the proteins are the cell component that make enzymes and do work, the genes will control what happens with the cells. At the very earliest time of development, there are a variety of genes that become active to direct all that needs to occur. First off, the single fertilized egg, now called a zygote, becomes a a group of many cells by dividing in half repeatedly. This creates a ball of cells about a week after fertilization. It is at this point (roughly a week after fertilization) that the zygote will implant in the lining of the uterus. Until then, it floats freely in the uterus, and after the implantation it will have access to the mother's blood supply to begin to absorb new nutrients so the zygote will be able to grow in size. This means the one original egg cell is the same total size as the ball of cells, but the ball of cells (called a blastocyst) has over 100 cells (this can happen because the egg cell is very large to start, so as it divides into hundreds of cells, these individual cells become much smaller, finally becoming the size of regular human cells).

At the time of implanting, the cells of the blastocyst are beginning to change. The change is a beginning of specializing, where each cell takes on certain functions and loses other functions. This specialization (called differentiation) begins due to the relative locations of the cells in the ball of cells (blastocyst). As this happens, the cells group into three layers, each with different characteristics. What is amazing is that the layers are not interchangeable. Once they have begun to specialize into one layer or another they cannot change, and this is because their genes effectively become locked for life. So, cells that will soon form the heart cannot form the brain. In this way, the patterns for developing organs is set at this very early time, and as the organs develop they can form in the correct locations because they start forming in these places. This wondrous dance of cells very early in development sets the stage for the accurate development of our entire body.

With these rapid changes and the fast pace of cells growing and moving into position, any perturbation can cause substantial problems. This is why exposure of a pregnant woman to various drugs or chemicals can change the way the fetal cells are functioning and thus create a different pattern of development. For this reason, it is advisable for a pregnant person to keep away from things that may not be absolutely safe. Any small change at this point in fetal life may have a profound effect as a small perturbation creates a different environment or a new pattern of development for the fetus. Indeed, even after a child is born, the rapid rate of cell division means that exposure to something that can change development can have a lasting impact on the child, and one that may not be reversible.

# Heart and Lungs

The heart, blood and blood vessels are called the cardiovascular system. Its function is to distribute things in the body. The things carried include the gases oxygen and carbon dioxide, which are exchanged with air in our lungs (taking in oxygen and getting rid of carbon dioxide), the nutrients from our foods that enter from the digestive system, the waste products from our organs that may be detoxified by the liver and then removed by the kidneys, the signaling molecules called hormones that control a lot of systems in the body, and illness fighting compounds like white blood cells and antibodies.

## *Blood*

The blood carries all of these components. Blood itself is made of the liquid part, called plasma, and the cells. The cells include red blood cells, which carry oxygen inside them, and modify carbon dioxide so it can be dissolved in the blood liquid; white blood cells, which are used to protect us from infection; and platelets, which are cell fragments and are used to plug a hole in a blood vessel and prevent blood loss. The liquid plasma makes up just over half of the total volume of the blood, with the red blood cells making up most of the rest (the white blood cells are a tiny fraction of the total). The plasma itself is much thicker than water due to all the proteins that it carries around. Some of these proteins are hormones, some are proteins that carry steroids and other fats, and there's a collection of proteins in our blood that are ready to make a blood clot when we have a damaged blood vessel. These proteins make the initial soft blood clot and then convert it into a hard one to make sure that when we have a punctured vessel we do not lose much blood. The most common blood protein is called albumin. Albumin is used to keep water in the blood by making blood thicker than water and in that way keeping up the liquid pressure. This let's blood carry a lot of different substances. You can get a sense for this by looking at egg white also has a lot of albumin, and also keeps a constant liquid pressure in the egg. Blood plasma also carries all the minerals and vitamins through our body, and is the delivery system for all of the food nutrients and water throughout the body.

### Blood Vessels

Blood is pumped by the heart and carried inside blood vessels. The heart generates pressure to push the blood throughout the body, so the vessels leaving the heart, called arteries, must hold this pressure in order for the blood to reach our hands and feet (called our extremities). Arteries are surrounded by a layer of smooth muscle that tightens around the artery to keep the pressure inside. This tightening of smooth muscle is called vasoconstriction, and its opposite is vasodilation (opening up, or dilating, the blood vessel). Vasoconstriction increases blood pressure. We use it when we are scared and we have an adrenalin rush, to force blood to quickly move to our muscles and run. We also use vasoconstriction to reduce blood flow to our extremities (hands and feet) when they are very cold (and hence why your hands are measurably colder when you feel cold; your body is decreasing blood flow to the areas far away to keep from losing too much body heat. There are also a lot of different drugs that stimulate vasoconstriction for a little while, including caffeine, antihistamines, and stimulants.

The arteries start with the largest artery, the aorta, which is

26

just over 25 mm (1 inch) in diameter and carries blood from the heart, directing it first upward (ascending aorta) and then curving downward (arch of the aorta and descending aorta). The major arteries branch off from the aorta and carry blood to all the organ systems of the body, branching into arterioles (small arteries) to direct blood to every part of every organ. Arterioles have small valves (a ring of smooth muscle called a sphincter that can clamp down and reduce blood flow), so it is the control of these sphincters that allows lets our body control the blood flow to the every tissue, bringing more or less blood as each area needs more or less oxygen.

Blood from the arterioles enters capillaries, the smallest blood vessels, which branch out in each area of tissue. We have a tremendous number of capillary beds, each receiving blood from an arteriole. The capillaries are thin, leaky vessels, allowing blood plasma to leak out into the surrounding tissue and provide it with nutrients, as well as remove wastes. The fluid leaking out does so because of the pressure that has moved blood all the way to the capillary. As the fluid is pushed out by the pressure, what stays behind inside the capillaries are the cells, because they are too large to leak out. As fluid leaves but larger things stay, this makes an osmotic pull (the higher number of cells in the blood liquid pulls more liquid back into the capillaries) to return fluid back to the capillary. This is not perfect, as more fluid leaves than returns, with most of the rest of the fluid retained with the lymphatic system of vessels.

Blood leaving the capillaries enters the veins, which are low-pressure vessels in our body. Veins carry blood back to the heart. The veins are more flexible than arteries, and they have internal one-way valves to make sure the blood can only flow back toward the heart. Coming from the capillaries are the venules (little veins), which combine to form veins, and these veins combine close to the heart into the vena cava. It is the vena cava that drains into the heart.

While pressure pushes plasma out of the capillaries, it is the increased concentration in the capillary from the decreased liquid that pulls the liquid back into it for the return to the heart. This allows new fluid to change with old fluid, bringing the needed oxygen and removing the carbon dioxide, but it also leaves behind a small amount of liquid outside of the blood vessels because the fluid pushed out by pressure is more than the fluid pulled in by osmosis. The extra plasma fluid that leaves the capillaries is picked up and returned to the heart by another fluid system in our bodies, the lymphatic system.

### Lymphatic vessels and lymph nodes

The lymphatic vessels (often called lymphatics for short) are a series of low-pressure veins, all of which have one-way valves inside so that the fluid will only flow back to the vena cava. In many ways, these lymphatics are like the blood veins, they are flexible, have valves and the fluid is at low pressure. However, they drain the excess fluid that can accumulate in all our tissues, and return it to the heart. Along the way through the body, these lymphatic 'veins' pass through lymph nodes. Lymph nodes filter the fluid in lymphatics and screen it for anything foreign that might infect our body. When something does enter our body, the immune system cells inside lymph nodes set up to attack and destroy this foreign danger, as we discuss in the immune system chapter.

### Veins and blood flow

All veins are at low pressure, while arteries are at high pressure. It is the pressure that moves blood through the arteries to the most distant points of the body. So what forces blood to return to the heart in veins? Part of this force is the blood moving and the one-way valves that keep it from ever going backward. But another way the blood flows back to the heart in our veins is the contraction of our muscles. Veins are stretchier than arteries, so more blood can be inside them since they can expand. Also, while arteries are deep below the skin, veins are near the surface (the expression used to refer to this is that arteries are deep and veins are superficial). This separation protects the arteries from injury. Indeed, if an artery is cut, blood comes out in pulses, while if a vein is cut the blood merely seeps out. In the artery case a person can lose a lot of blood quickly while in the vein case, the blood loss may be minimal, and further loss is prevented by a platelet forming a plug in the break of the vein, while a clot begins to form to allow the vein to heal.

With the low pressure inside veins, every time you contract a muscle next to a vein, that pushes on the soft vein, pushing on the blood inside it. Because of the one-way valves inside the veins, this pushed blood can only move toward the heart. This additional blood movement increases the blood moving back to the heart when you move your legs or arms, or even when you stand. This simple action means that as soon as you start moving, you instantly increase the flow of your blood (allowing more oxygen to be sent around to your muscles to help them make energy for that movement). This automatic mechanism is referred to as a skeletal muscle pump, because the muscle that pushes on the vein is the same muscle that is attached to our bones (the skeleton)..

### Heart

The strong pump that moves blood through the arteries is the heart. Our heart is really a pair of pumps that are side-by-side, one on the left side of the heart and the other on the right, each of which has two chambers. The size of your heart is roughly the size of your fist, and if you make a fist with your right hand and hold it up against the left side of your chest, as though you were covering your left breast but with your fist, you have the idea of both the size and approximate location of your heart.

The role of the heart is to pump blood through two different circulatory systems. A circulatory system is a system of arteries, capillaries and veins that makes a circle. One circle pumps blood that is low in oxygen to the lungs to get oxygenated and then return to the heart, while the other circle pumps the blood to all the parts of the body, delivering that oxygen to all our tissues and organs. The first system is called the pulmonary circulation (meaning that it goes to the lungs) and the second is called the systemic circulation (because it goes to all the organ systems in the body).

### Blood flow in the heart

Let's follow the movement of blood through the heart, starting with the flow entering the heart from the body by way of the vena cava. The vena cava is carrying blood that is lower in oxygen since it is returning from the body's systems. This blood enters the top of the right side of the heart, arriving first into the top heart chamber called the right atrium. When the atrium beats, that pushes the blood inside it into the right ventricle (the heart chamber just below the atrium). To enter the right ventricle, the blood flows through a one-way valve that separates the atrium from the ventricle. This valve is called an atrio-ventricular valve (this particular AV valve is called the tricuspid valve). When the right ventricle beats, the blood is forced out of the ventricle, passing through a valve (called a semi-lunar valve because it looks like two half-moons) and into the pulmonary artery to travel to the lungs. At the lungs, carbon dioxide is leaves the blood and oxygen is absorbed into the blood. The oxygen gets stored inside the red blood cells bound to molecules containing iron that are called hemoglobin. This oxygenated blood then flows back to the heart through the pulmonary vein, entering into the left atrium.

When the left atrium beats, it pushes the oxygenated blood into the left ventricle (through an AV valve called the mitral valve). When the left ventricle beats, it squeezes the blood out through a semi-lunar valve into the aorta to begin flowing through the systemic circulation.

Overall, blood flows into the heart by entering the atria and leaves the heart from the ventricles. This means the ventricles are the stronger of the two chambers, with the atria responsible for about 20 percent of the pumping and the ventricles handling all the rest of the work. The right side of the heart has the blood lower in oxygen and sends it to the lungs, while the left side of the heart handles the oxygenated blood and sending it to the entire body. Since the lungs are very close to the heart, this means the right side of the heart does not need the strength that the left side does. But the left ventricle, which pushes the blood to all the systems, is much thicker than the right and therefore much stronger than it. The left side of the heart needs this additional strength to pump blood all the way to the extremities. The result is that the pressure of the blood leaving the left ventricle is higher than the pressure from the right side. Blood pressure measurements tell what this pressure is in the arteries. These measurements have two numbers, high pressure (systole) over low pressure (diastole). Systole occurs when the ventricle contracts, while diastole occurs when the ventricle relaxes.

*Heart muscle*

The heart is made of a type of muscle called cardiac muscle. This is one of the three types of muscle in our bodies, and cardiac muscle is only found in the heart. The other two types of muscle are smooth muscle, which surrounds hollow internal organs (like the smooth muscle that is around our digestive tract to push the foods along) and skeletal muscle, which connects to the bones (the skeleton) and moves our body. Skeletal and cardiac muscle have a striped appearance due to the array of contractile proteins stacked inside these muscle cells, while smooth muscle has an even texture as the proteins are oriented in multiple directions. While cardiac and skeletal muscles are similar in strength and in how they contract, cardiac muscle has two unique features: all the cardiac cells are electrically and physically connected to each other, and the cardiac muscle cells have a longer period of contraction than skeletal muscle to be able to push the blood out with each contraction.

The electrical coupling of cardiac muscle cells makes the heart operate like one unit, when one cell in the atrium is stimulated to contract, all the cells throughout the two atria receive this electrical stimulation. The physical coupling of the cardiac cells results in each contraction pulling the whole muscle, so that it collapses in like a balloon collapses in when air is released from it.

When one part of the atrium is electrically stimulated, the entire atrium contracts. This stimulation gets to the ventricles with a short delay (about a tenth of a second), so they contract in the same fashion as the atria, collapsing inward to push the blood from the ventricles and send it into the arteries.

While all the cells of the heart are electrically excitable, there is a specialized area in the right atrium to set the pace. This pacemaker of the heart is in the sinoatrial node (SA node). The SA node is rhythmically contractile, meaning that it creates an electrical pulse about once a second that is sent through the electrical coupling to all the atrial cells. The SA node can speed up or slow down our heartrate by control from our brain. In this way, our brain can increase our heartrate when we are active and using more oxygen and slow it down when we are at rest.

The other unique feature of cardiac muscle is the longer period of contraction for each electrical pulse. In skeletal muscle, when we contract the muscle, each pulse has a very small effect, and it is only when we have a lot of pulses that we get the strong contraction we are familiar with to lift things. In the heart we never have a strong sustained contraction that we do with our arms or legs, but each individual contracting pulse lasts for about two tenths of a second. This relatively long pulse is enough to allow all the cells of the atria or all the cells of the ventricles to contract inward, and eject all the blood inside the chamber.

## *Electrocardiograph (ECG or EKG)*

Because all cardiac muscle cells work as one, and because the contraction is caused by movement of the electrical stimulation, we can measure the electrical activity of the heart by measuring the electrocardiogram, called briefly the ECG or EKG. The ECG has a few waves when recorded, with each being related to a heart chamber. The first wave is the P wave and it is from the electrical stimulation of the atria that causes them to contract. So the P wave is the atrial contraction. The biggest wave is called the QRS complex, and this is when the ventricles contract. The last wave is the T wave, and this is when the ventricles relax (their charge is repolarized and they relax). Since the ventricles are contracting from the QRS to the T wave, during this time the heart is at high pressure (systole), while it is at low pressure (diastole) when the ventricles are relaxing (from T to the next QRS).

## *Heart sounds*

The heartbeat that we hear from our hearts (the lub-dub sound) is called the heart sounds, with the first heart sound and second heart sound being the ones we are can hear when we rest our head on our pillow and hear our heart. These sounds are made by the closing of the two sets of valves in the heart. The first heart sound is from the closing of the AV valves, which occurs when the ventricles start to contract. The second heart sound is from the closing of the semilunar valves, which occurs when the ventricles begin to relax. Because the contraction and relaxation of the ventricle is synchronized with the ECG, the first heart sound happens during the QRS complex, while the second heart sound occurs with the T wave.

A common measure of heart function is the cardiac output. Cardiac output is the amount of blood pumped by the heart per minute. It is equal to the number of heart beats per minute (the heart rate) times the amount of blood leaving from the ventricle per beat of the heart (called the stroke volume). Cardiologists refer to this cardiac output as being equal to stroke volume times heart rate. Since the stroke volume is affected by the amount of blood coming into the heart from the vena cava (recall that when we move this increases the blood returning to the heart), then the stroke volume is directly related to this venous return. Since cardiac output is a measure of the heart activity, some diagnostic tests use this cardiac output measurement during various levels of exercise to determine the strength of a person's heart and relate their cardiac output to what the typical person measure may have. If someone has had a heart attack, often their cardiac output is reduced from normal, which limits how much strenuous activity they can do.

Even when we are fully resting, our cardiac output rarely goes below 20 percent, as our brain uses 15 percent or more of the heart's output, while the heart itself needs another 3 percent or 4 percent. The part of the body that has the biggest range of blood use are the skeletal muscles, which use up to 70 percent of the blood pumped by the heart each minute when we exercise vigorously.

*Lungs*

The work of our lungs is to exchange gases with the air around us. When we breath in, our lungs are filled with air that has normal levels of oxygen and carbon dioxide, and when we breath out, we push out air that has lower amounts of oxygen and higher amounts of carbon dioxide. The reason is that we use oxygen to help provide energy for all the cells in our body, and the waste product from this energy production is carbon dioxide. We constantly replace the oxygen and get rid of the carbon dioxide. The process of moving oxygen in and out of the body is called respiration (in a similar way, the process of moving oxygen into and out of each cell is called cellular respiration). So, respiratory function is to bring air in (called inspiration or inhalation) and expel air (called expiration or exhalation).

Both oxygen and carbon dioxide are gases, and cannot stay dissolved in blood very long. To recognize this, realize what happens when you blow air underwater, the bubbles rise up to return to the air. A small amount will dissolve in the water, but most will return to the air above. In order for our bodies to carry enough oxygen to our cells, we have specialized cells called red blood cells, or erythrocytes, that have molecules of hemoglobin inside them. The function of red blood cells is to carry oxygen, and they do so using the hemoglobin, which holds the oxygen so that it can stay in the blood and not create bubbles. Almost all (99 percent) of the oxygen in our body is carried by hemoglobin. As the red blood cells travel through the blood, they release some oxygen in areas that are low in oxygen. This oxygen travels the short distance to the cells needing oxygen by diffusion. Similarly, as carbon dioxide is made by these same body cells, it diffuses into the blood and the same red blood cells convert it into a form that can dissolve in the blood. This form is called bicarbonate. Bicarbonate is made from carbon dioxide and water, and it is used by our blood to help control the acidity of the blood. This means that carbon dioxide is buffering the acidity, and so it is called a buffer for pH (pH is a measure of acidity, with a pH of 7 being neutral, lower numbers being acidic and higher numbers being alkaline).

One other challenge in getting a gas into the blood is that it has to first dissolve into liquid before it can be absorbed into the body. Since only a very small amount of oxygen can dissolve in water, we need a large area to collect enough oxygen to power our body. Our lungs are designed to fill with air when we take a breath. As the air moves in, it flows down our trachea (in our neck) and into our bronchi (at the top of our chest). The bronchi are large tubes that allow the air to flow into the lobes of the lungs. The bronchi branch into smaller tubes called bronchioles, which end in tiny sacs called alveoli. The alveoli are packed along the bronchioles like clusters of grapes, except they are much smaller. Each alveolus is about 4 micrometers (a micrometer is one thousandth of a millimeter) in diameter, and an adult has about a half billion alveoli. A measure of the number of alveoli in each cubic millimeter of lung found it to be around 170. This puts estimates of the total surface area of all the alveoli in our lungs at approximately 100 square meters, the size of an 1100 sf apartment! This immense area is packed inside our chest in the lungs, and we need it to absorb enough oxygen each minute to keep all the cells in the body supplied.

One other critical lung feature that allows oxygen to dissolve is that the entire inside lining of the alveoli and bronchioles is coated with a thin film of liquid. This liquid is secreted by the lungs, and contains mucus and a surfactant. The mucus is to catch dust along the way into the lungs to make sure it does not get stuck in the alveoli and cause irritation that harms our breathing. The surfactant is like a soapy coating, and keeps the alveoli slippery. When we breathe out, we expel air from the alveoli and the alveoli linings. By having surfactant coating the inner lining of the alveoli, this thin tissue cannot stick together, much as when your hands are soapy and they slide freely against each other.

The mucus is continually moved back up the airways (the bronchioles and bronchi and trachea), and into the pharynx of the upper throat. From here we clear it out by coughing. This keeps the lungs clear of debris that would otherwise irritate the thin alveoli and cause damage to them. Indeed, people exposed to extensive fine dust will have particles of it get through and lodge inside their lungs, which can inflame the tissue and reduce respiratory function. This is the case for individuals who smoke or live or work in areas with soot. The inflammation caused by the smoke or soot staying in their lungs irritates the lining of the lungs and this can cause mutations that lead to cancer (see chapter on cancer). The same particles in the lungs can diminish respiratory ability of the lungs, making it more difficult to bring in sufficient amounts of oxygen for the body.

Lung infection from a virus can also hurt respiration, as the lungs will increase their secretions. This increase in mucus will help catch anything coming in through the airways, but the increased liquid results in more fluid inside the lungs. The thicker layer of liquid means that it will take a little longer for each oxygen to diffuse into the blood, and someone in this situation will feel a shortness of breath that improves itself as they return to health from the illness. Because we are always breathing in the air around us, the lungs have a strong immune system response to protect us from infection (see immune system chapter). We constantly attack any foreign microbe that gets in to keep it from infecting us.

The lung fluids are in a constantly being made by the lungs, being expelled to clear the dust and being absorbed into the blood. The absorption also occurs in the alveoli. The thin layer of fluid that the oxygen dissolves into is pulled by the movement of blood around the alveoli back into the capillaries surrounding the alveoli. This fluid movement provides the pulling force to move lung fluid into the blood fluid. The constant production of lung fluid is in balance with the constant removal of this fluid, keeping the body oxygenated, and the lungs clear. When the fluid is not pulled out fast enough, as explained below in congestive heart failure, the fluid causes lung congestion that slows down our oxygen intake, limiting our energy and how much we can do.

# HEART AND BLOOD VESSEL DISORDERS

There are a number of health conditions that affect the heart and blood vessels (this combination of heart and blood vessels is called the cardiovascular system). In fact, there are a lot of common heart and blood vessel conditions. Damage to the cardiovascular system is the most common chronic medical condition seen in the developed world and is increasingly common in the developing world. These conditions arise from lifestyle choices and from family history. Another way to say this is that these conditions arise from diet and exercise as well as from the genes we each inherit. We know that certain diets are beneficial and other diets are damaging, and we know that exercise is almost always beneficial.

## Blood Vessels

While there are genetic conditions that increase one's risk for plaque buildup inside the arteries, it seems that the majority of people with higher levels of arterial plaque have it due to the consumption of foods with higher cholesterol content in conjunction with low exercise levels. Hypercholesterolemia, or high cholesterol in the blood, is the term given to these conditions. One type of this disease, familial hypercholesterolemia, is genetic and so is passed down in families. People with diabetes or with a thyroid gland that is under-active (i.e., low hormone secretion) may also have high cholesterol levels. But most people with high cholesterol have it due to diet. In these diet-caused cases, it seems that the issue is not the consumption of cholesterol itself, but which type of cholesterol is consumed. Cholesterol is a lipid (a hydrocarbon, or oil) and so cannot dissolve in water. Since blood is a water-based liquid, cholesterol does not dissolve in it, and must be carried in the blood by proteins called lipoproteins. All lipids in the blood have carrier proteins to shuttle them around to where they are needed. And since every cell in our body uses lipids to keep the cell intact, these lipids are needed throughout the body. Cholesterol is categorized by its density when it is attached to the lipoprotein. Thus we have cholesterol attached to high density lipoprotein (HDL) or low density lipoprotein (LDL) or others (such as very low density).

We know that LDL (and lower density lipoproteins) are the type that increase our risk and HDL decrease our risk for cardiovascular disease. This means increased risk is related to increase in non-HDL cholesterol. A good way to reduce our risk is to consume more fiber (the LDL cholesterol sticks to it and is removed), reduce saturated fat and trans fat in the food you eat, and use non-saturated fats. Additionally, it is important to be physically active (which helps the body use more of the cholesterol so that it does not build up as much). Some people find that eating more plants and less meat is helpful, as plants provide fiber and help decrease saturated fats. Overall, saturated fats are found in animals, while plants do not make cholesterol and only have unsaturated fats. There may also be a benefit to consuming plant-based sterols (phytosterols) in lowering LDL. Eliminating trans fats (which are artificially produced from vegetable fat) in the diet is certainly beneficial as our body does not process these well and they raise our risk for heart disease by increasing LDL and decreasing HDL. Replacing saturated fats with mono-unsaturated fats (such as olive oil) or poly-unsaturated fats seems to provide the greatest benefit, and current studies indicate a Mediterranean diet, which has lots of vegetables and fruits as well as fish, and uses olive oil as the primary fat, is helpful for most people.

## High Blood Pressure - Hypertension

When there is a lot of LDL cholesterol, it can stick to the inside of arteries in what is called plaque. As plaque develops inside the arteries, it shrinks the room for the blood to travel. The same volume of blood still needs to get through these arteries, and so the heart pumps a little harder to provide enough force to push the same amount of blood. The result is that someone with plaque lining the arteries develops higher blood pressure because of these small openings. High blood pressure, called hypertension, can damage blood vessels.

The best treatment for hypertension due to vascular problems like plaque is modifying our diet and increasing exercise to reduce the plaque buildup. This is a slow process as it involves lifestyle changes, but it typically has good results in terms of not only the immediate problem (the hypertension) but in improving the quality of life overall. Appropriate diets and exercise are discussed in later chapters.

## Coronary Artery Blockage

If there is plaque inside the arteries that provide oxygen to the heart itself, this can cause severe problems. The arteries that provide oxygen to the heart are called coronary arteries and they branch off the aorta to go directly to the heart muscle and provide it the oxygen it needs to function. These vessels are called coronary arteries because they circle the heart like a crown. Without them, the heart muscle cannot get the constant supply of oxygen and glucose it needs to keep pumping (the blood inside the heart doesn't reach into the heart muscle to provide oxygen, but capillaries attached to the coronary arteries do). If any coronary artery has a lot of plaque, the pressure in that artery goes up and less blood and oxygen reaches the heart muscle. A decrease in blood to the heart muscle is a problem, because the heart is always ready to beat faster when we get active. If a coronary artery has a block, that part of the heart will not get enough oxygen when the heart needs to beat faster. This means the heart will be starved of oxygen when it's needed, and there can be damage.

Treatment for a blocked artery can take several forms. If it is not severe, lifestyle changes can be helpful, using is a change in diet and increase in exercise to gradually make improvement. The next step up is a simple surgical action like angioplasty, when a balloon catheter is used to flatten the plaque inside the artery and make a more open passage, or a stent is placed inside to hold the artery open. More major surgery can involve a bypass, where the blocked artery is replaced with a leg vein from the patient to allow blood to pass through.

### Aortic Aneurysm

An aortic aneurysm is a swelling of the aorta such that the wall of the aorta balloons outward, looking like a swollen tube. Aneurysms can occur on the aorta in the chest (called Thoracic Aortic Aneurysm) or in the abdomen or gut (called Abdominal Aortic Aneurysm). An aneurysm can be life threatening if it ruptures, as a person would rapidly bleed inside their body from the largest artery. Aneurysms typically affect people over 65 who have a family history of them, or who smoke or have hardening of the arteries or a history of drug use or a traumatic injury to the area. They also afflict men more than women. Since there are no strong symptoms of them, people with multiple risk factors should be screened with ultrasound imaging to determine if there is an aneurysm developing. If there is an aneurysm over 5 cm, it can be treated surgically with a graft.

In contrast to aortic aneurysms, cerebral aneurysms (swelling of a blood vessel in the brain) occur more frequently in women, and there are more symptoms as the aneurysm pushes onto a brain structure. Some of these symptoms include loss of balance or perception, speech problems or double vision, or fatigue. Treatment often involves minimal surgical intervention.

## Heart Attack

If part of the heart is starved for oxygen, this can cause a myocardial infarction (MI), more commonly known as a heart attack. An MI occurs in the part of the heart that is starved for oxygen. When the heart needs to beat harder, this area does not receive enough blood for it to do so and the muscle cells essentially starve to death. From that point on, this damaged area of the heart can no longer contract, and the heart's pumping becomes less effective as this inactive bit of muscle stretches and becomes less effective, decreasing the overall cardiac output.

An MI can occur in any part of the heart, and the location of it and the size of it will determine how big an effect it has. An MI in each chamber of the heart has different effects. If the MI is in one of the atria, it usually has the smallest effect on the heart's cardiac output because the atria only contribute about 20 percent of the total cardiac output. An MI in the left atrium, for example, may reduce the maximal output by as much as 20 percent, though an MI in the right atrium could have a more serious effect if it occurs at the heart's pacemaker.

## Pacemaker

The pacemaker of the heart is in the right atrium in the SA node. If the SA node is damaged in a myocardial infarction, the pacemaker may no longer function to pace the heart. Fortunately, all heart muscle cells are rhythmically contractile, meaning they will contract on their own if there is no pacesetter. But their natural rate of contraction is slower than our normal rate (about 40-60 beats per minute). Additionally, it is only the pacemaker that can change the heart rhythm, so if it doesn't work, the person's heart cannot speed up with activity. This problem is treated now by inserting an electronic pacemaker to pace the heart, with a control that the recipient can use to increase or decrease their heartrate. The electronic pacemaker allows someone to function normally, increasing their heart rate when more active, decreasing it when less active.

## Valves

Sometimes an MI occurs around one of the valves. In this case, the area around the valve becomes floppier, and the sides of the valve spread apart, leaving a gap between them. This looks like a door that is too small for its opening, and the door flops back and forth. it doesn't matter which valve gets floppy, the result is inefficient pumping of blood and a big decrease in cardiac output. If we cannot find a way to tighten the heart muscle around the valve, the most common solution is to surgically remove the valve and replace it with a mechanical valve or the valve from the heart of a pig that has been treated to be neutral in the human body (essentially sterilized so that there are no pig proteins visible to our immune system). Why is a pig heart used? Pig hearts are very similar to human hearts in their size and function, and the valves work well as replacements.

## Fibrillation

If the heart muscle is sufficiently irritated by the damage, we often see a problem called fibrillation. Fibrillation is when the muscle tries to contract hundreds of times a minute, looking almost like it is shivering. This problem arises when there is a damaged area in the heart and a wave of stimulation circles around, stimulating the same cells over and over several times a second. This rapid series of very brief contractions means the heart cells cannot contract all the way, so the blood cannot fully leave the heart chambers. This can be a life-threatening situation. It usually occurs after a heart attack, when the heart is irritated by the damage and the heart cells are weakened overall, causing them to be easy to over stimulate. If the damaged area is in the ventricles, immediate attention is critical for survival. With ventricular fibrillation, the cardiac output drops precipitously, as the heart never fully ejects the blood in the ventricle, so not enough blood circulates. In this situation, it is urgent to try to reset the heart rhythm. This can be done with an electrical pulse through a defibrillator, and for this reason these devices have become common in work sites. It is also possible to reset the cardiac rhythm with a swift physical shock to the chest above the heart. This latter method is often successful for those trained in it, and it is done by forcefully slapping the chest with an open palm. If you feel it is necessary to use this method, strike hard enough to create a pressure pulse that will possibly reset the heart but not so hard that you may break a bone.

Atrial fibrillation is when the damage is in the atrium and the top part of the heart fibrillates. While dangerous and requiring treatment, it is not as devastating as ventricular fibrillation. Since the atria are responsible for 20 percent of the cardiac output, with atrial fibrillation, a person still has 80 percent of their cardiac output. Atrial fibrillation can be best treated by bringing someone to medical care where they can monitor and choose the optimal course of action. Medical personnel will be able to choose the right action, which may involve several things to calm the heart and stop the fibrillation.

### Congestive Heart Failure

When someone has substantially reduced cardiac output, they can be at risk for congestive heart failure. And while the name of this condition sounds particularly ominous when you first hear it, most people diagnosed with congestive heart failure live for many years with it. The words "heart failure" sounds frightening, of course, but the reality is that the name of this condition is about the congestion and its cause. Congestive heart failure is a medical condition where the lungs are congested, and this congestion is because of a decrease in cardiac output. Most often, this decreased cardiac output is due to a heart attack, where the heart is no longer able to contract as strongly as it used to. Because of the weaker contractions, blood is pumped out from the heart at a slower speed. To understand why there is congestion from a decreased output, we need to recall how the lungs work. There is fluid inside the lungs to allow the oxygen to dissolve and to keep the lining of the lungs from sticking together. This fluid is constantly being made and constantly being removed. Its removal is automatic, pulled out by the fast moving blood around each of the alveoli. The blood movement creates a suction to pull fluid out of the alveoli.

When blood moves slower, the suction for the fluid in the lungs is also decreased, and fluid can build up inside the lungs. If fluid builds up in the lungs, then it takes longer for oxygen to diffuse through this fluid and get to the blood. The result is a person will be starved for air even while breathing normally, as the air they breathe in takes longer to get through the thick layer of fluid in the alveoli. This person will usually wheeze while breathing and feel that it is hard to breath in. One of the exercises to counter this is to take deep breaths. A useful treatment currently is for the person to take a diuretic. A diuretic is a drug that makes a person urinate more than. If someone with lung congestion urinates more, it makes their blood slightly more concentrated, which helps to pull more water out of the lungs and clear them of the excess fluid.

People with congestive heart failure usually need to be less active because of the lower cardiac output, and it takes more effort for them to do things, since their ability to get oxygen into the blood is slower. Another observation is that their ankles and wrists are usually swollen. This is for the same reason as the fluid building up in the lungs, the slower moving blood does not pull all the fluid back into the veins, and so a little is left behind in their arms and legs. Congestive heart failure is treated as a chronic (i.e., long-term) disease, so medications to increase the heart's contractibility and to increase urination are used to alleviate the condition. Additionally, deep breathing exercises and movements such as walking are used to help move the fluid and help it clear from the lungs.

## Heart Sounds

Often, people will learn that they have a heart sound. A heart sound is a very general term to mean any sound that is coming from the area of the heart. There are many things that can create sounds in the heart, with the most obvious being the heartbeat sound made from the closing of the AV valves and semilunar valves. These are normal sounds that everyone has. There are other heart sounds that are normal, but difficult to hear, but there are sounds that have more concern, and these are informative to a trained physician. Some sound like clicks, and these are usually valves that are a bit sticky. Occasionally, someone will have a whoosh sound from their heart and this can mean that a valve is letting blood go through it in the reverse direction, perhaps because the valve does not close fully. Sometimes a person may have a small perforation between the left and right atria (a "hole" in their heart), in which case the blood with oxygen and the blood that is low in oxygen mix a bit. This is more common in newborns who are premature, and the reason is that the atria do not separate fully into right and left until after we are born. If they do not close on their own, it is possible to surgically go in and close them, but usually they seal without such action. For a baby, if the opening is small enough, the risk is low, particularly if it will seal on its own, so surgery is not the first choice unless there are other concerns.

If you are told you have a heart sound, a plan is to ask

questions so you understand what makes the sound and what it means for you. The questions are: What is making the sound (be sure to ask a follow up to clarify if you did not understand); how concerned should I be – am I at risk for anything and when may that happen?; should I change my activities because of this?; what should I watch for that means I should come in for an exam?

# Digestion

We need to eat to get the nutrients and energy we need each day. The nutrients are called major nutrients and minor nutrients. The major nutrients are things we need a lot of each day, such as protein, carbohydrates, fats and water. The minor nutrients are ones we only need a little bit of, such as vitamins and minerals. Both major and minor nutrients are needed each day, and our digestive system takes these foods, breaks them into their building blocks, and then absorbs these subunits into our blood.

Overall, the minor nutrients are from food, and we absorb them into our blood. The major nutrients have a two-step process to be absorbed. Because they are large molecules, they first must be broken down into their subunits (the building blocks for the carbs, protein and fats), and then they can be absorbed. For carbohydrates, this means being broken into sugars. Fats are broken into fatty acids and glycerol, and proteins are split into amino acid. Our gut can absorb these small molecules, but it cannot absorb the larger ones. If we did not break down the carbohydrates or fats or protein, they would pass through our digestive system and be eliminated. So we need to break apart the foods to use the nutrients.

Once these foods are broken down, they travel in our blood and are picked up by cells to use for building new molecules. Each cell is a small factory, constantly making proteins and membrane and energy and signal molecules. To make these molecules, the cell needs a constant supply of the raw materials, in the form of sugars, fatty acids, amino acids, vitamins and minerals.

In fact, all living things need sugars, amino acids and fatty acids to make their cells. This is because all living things have a similar structure, being made of cells, using proteins to do work, carbohydrates and fats to provide energy and structure. For all cells, the sugars, amino acids and fatty acids are the molecular building blocks necessary to make the bigger molecules that the cells need. All animals eat these nutrients to get the building blocks, but plants are able to make their sugars directly from sunlight, carbon dioxide and water. Because plants make the energy they need, they are self-sufficient. They still need to absorb minerals, but they make the energy and molecules that we and all animals need to eat to survival.

## Digestive System

Our digestive system has several organs that work together to break down the food products we consume, absorb them into our blood and regulate the amount of each in our blood by storing molecules that can be used later. The organs are the gastrointestinal tract, liver, pancreas and gall bladder.

The gastrointestinal tract (GI tract) is a tube that goes through our body, starting at the mouth, going down to the stomach and intestines and exiting with the anus. Anything that crosses this GI tract gets inside the body (is absorbed) and anything that does not cross it, technically never enters the body, it stays in the tract and is eliminated in our feces. The tract has activity that allows digestion or absorption to take place, and these activities change as we move from one part of the GI tract to the next.

Functionally, the GI tract needs to break down the large molecules so they can be absorbed. To do this, several mechanical and chemical processes are used, with each one occurring in a different section of the tract. It all starts in the mouth, where our teeth chew the bites of food to break them into smaller particles. As we chew our food we secrete saliva to moisten it for swallowing and allow us to taste it more fully. Saliva contains an enzyme called amylase, which breaks down carbohydrate molecules into sugars. This is why starchy foods have a fuller taste as you chew them more, the amylase breaks off sugar groups that your tongue can then detect. Note that the foods do not taste sugary, they just increase their flavor as you chew and release some sugars to give more flavor.

Our tongues can detect at least five tastes: salt, sugar, sour, bitter and umami (delightful). We also have sensation of heat and cool, which respond to both temperature and hot pepper (heat) or menthol (cool), and there is some indication we may also sense fat. But foods taste many more flavors than these, and that is because our sense of smell gives important information for us as to what a food tastes like. Once we are chewing foods in our mouth, it is not only the taste buds on the tongue that detect the flavors in the food, there are many air-borne parts of the food that reach our olfactory sense in the area above our mouth and behind our nose, and this adds to our sense of the flavor of the food.

Saliva also contains mucus. Mucus is slippery and it coats foods they can slide along the GI tract without scratching. This is especially important for food we just put in our mouth, as it can be dry, and our esophagus (the part of the GI tract that connects from below the mouth to the stomach) needs to be protected from scratching. Anytime you swallow without chewing, or you take a bite of food that is too large, you may experience the discomfort of feeling it scratch its way down to your stomach. That is because food not coated with mucus scratches the esophagus. Also, when we drink liquids that are too hot, we risk scalding our throat or even our esophagus.

Scratching and scalding, if they occur regularly, can cause inflammation (irritation) of these areas, which increase our risk of developing cancer in those particular areas, as is discussed in the cancer chapter. In general, if it hurts, it is inflaming the area, and if this happens often, it may mutate some cells in the region and make them pre-cancerous.

Once we swallow, the food moves along our esophagus by peristalsis to go to our stomach. Since peristalsis moves the food, we do not rely on gravity to move it, and we can be lying down or weightless while eating and the food will still travel to our stomach.

### Stomach

The stomach is a unique environment in our body. It has an extra layer of smooth muscle around it so that it can mix its contents very well. It has a sphincter (this is a ring of muscle that clamps down on the GI tract to stop the flow) on each end to keep the contents contained in the stomach. Once food from a meal enters the stomach it stays there for a while and becomes well mixed with the stomach secretions.

The secretions from the stomach are mucus (a thick layer of mucus protects the lining of the stomach), an acid called hydrochloric acid, and an enzyme called pepsin. Pepsin is the only enzyme in our body that works in an acidic environment, and our stomach is very acidic, with a pH measure of 2 or 3 (pH is a measure of hydrogen ion, or acidity, and pH numbers less than 7 are acidic, with values below 4 very acidic). This level of acid is seen in a number of drinks, with most colas being around 3 and many citrus juices close to that level of acid.

Some people get heartburn, which is reflux of stomach contents into the esophagus due to a weak sphincter or to a large volume in the stomach. This burning feeling in the esophagus does not affect the heart but is called heartburn because the pain is felt near the heart. For those who often have stomach acids reach their mouth (either from reflux or from vomiting) or who consume a lot of acidic foods (such as cola or citrus), the enamel of their teeth will be eroded by this acid. Some enamel erosion happens from long term wear, but it is accelerated with acidic food/drink. If this is becoming a concern for you, it may be wise to reduce cola consumption, drink plain water after eating anything acidic, and waiting at least 20 minutes after these foods before brushing teeth so as not to scrub the enamel when it has been softened by acid.

The acidity of the stomach is for a very specific purpose. Among the food we eat, protein molecules are very long and they twist and coil on themselves to form tight 3-D structures in their natural form. With all the folding and twisting, it is difficult to use an enzyme to cut up the protein. By exposing the protein to acid, the coiling of the protein is relaxed and the protein strands straighten out. This relaxing of the natural shape is called denaturing the protein. Once this happens, the enzyme pepsin can chop the protein into smaller segments, called peptides.

Once food is well mixed in the stomach with the acid and enzyme, the protein will begin to break down. The stomach is good at mixing foods because of its extra layer of muscle. And the churning of the stomach begins when we eat, or when we think of food, or when we drink some alcohol. If the stomach is empty when this begins, we often hear the movement of air inside the stomach, a sound we call stomach "growling." It is simply that as we prepare for food, our stomach secretes the mucus and digestive fluids and starts mixing. If there is only some air and the mucus, the air bubble will mix back and forth and we hear it be pushed from one end of the stomach to the other, hearing it when we are hungry and just beginning to think of food.

*Intestine*

Once the stomach has finished breaking apart the proteins, the pyloric sphincter, the one that keeps food from leaving the stomach, relaxes and the stomach contents empty into the small intestine. Since these contents are acidic, our body immediately neutralizes the acid with buffers so we do not damage our intestine. These buffers are made by the pancreas and placed into the very first part of the small intestine (the duodenum). Along with buffers, the pancreas also makes a lot of enzymes that are used to break down all the food products. We have enzymes to cut up all the carbohydrate, protein, fat and nucleic acid (DNA) in the duodenum.

For the fats to break down, we need to let them mix first. Remember that oil and water do not normally mix. The liquid containing all the broken-down foods is primarily watery, so the fats in our food would stick together and not be digested unless we emulsify them. Emulsification is the process of allowing fats to mix with water. For example, soap emulsifies fat. When you wash an oily pan with soap, one side of the soap molecules surround each bit of fat and the other side of the soap molecules connect with the water. This means soap is amphipathic (meaning it likes both sides). It has two sides to it, and it can connect to both fat and water.

The compound our body makes to emulsify fats is bile. Bile is made by the liver and is stored in the gall bladder, a small sac that sits on the front surface of the liver. When fats enter the intestine, the gall bladder contracts to squeeze bile into the duodenum where it emulsifies the fats coming in. Once fat is emulsified, the enzymes can break it down into its component parts, which will be absorbed by the body.

*Nutrient Absorption*

Once the large molecules are broken down into their component pieces, these get absorbed into the blood along with the minerals and vitamins. Everything that dissolves in water goes right into a blood vessel that immediately travels to the liver, where most of the nutrients are removed and stored. Our liver provides a warehouse of nutrients that can then be slowly released all day so that our blood always has a supply of each nutrient. Because of its important role in storing nutrients, the liver of any animal is a nutrient-rich part of the body. This is why the color and taste of animal liver is intense, there are many vitamins and minerals and other nutrients in it.

Nutrients are absorbed along most of the small intestine. The large intestine absorbs water, and it packages the remaining wastes for elimination. The large intestine also harbors beneficial bacteria that eat some of the contents to synthesize vitamin B12 for us (which our body then absorbs and uses).

## Microbiome

We are learning that the good bacteria in our intestines, called the microbiome, are important to our health. For one, these good bacteria keep our gut healthy, and even make some things our body needs. When we get sick from food poisoning, our intestines empty out to remove the infection, but they hold a little of the good bacteria for when we are well. Also, eating cultured foods like yogurt, that has live bacterial cultures in it, helps keep a good balance of bacteria in our GI tract.

When a baby is born, it picks up these bacteria from its mother, and possibly also gets them from the first time nursing, when the baby drinks the colostrum (the first milk from the mother).

## Removal of wastes

In addition to bringing in new nutrients, we also need to remove wastes. In the digestive system, the non-digested materials are packaged in the colon for elimination. When we consume a lot of fiber (mostly vegetables and fruits), the fiber makes our waste material pack loosely, holding more water, and it is eliminated easily in a bowel movement. When we have very little fiber in our diet, the wastes are packed more solidly and move less readily. Additionally, the colon continues to absorb water out of the contents, so the wastes get packed a bit more tightly with time. Of course, the bacteria in our gut has more time to work on the wastes, making some nutrients for us (for example, vitamin K, which is needed for blood coagulation, is synthesized by microbes in our intestine).

In addition to the wastes from digestion, we also produce wastes within our body that need to be removed. These wastes are carbon dioxide, made in our cells when we use oxygen, as well as nitrogen containing waste that is a byproduct of our use of protein.

Carbon dioxide is removed primarily by the lungs, when we exhale it and inhale fresh oxygen for our blood. Our lungs can also help remove some of the acid in our body by getting rid of carbon dioxide, as we saw in the section on lungs. But more of the acid, along with the excess nitrogen, are removed by the kidneys. Our kidneys constantly filter the blood, and in the process remove excess nitrogen and acid, along with salt and water. While doing this, the kidneys save all the blood sugar for use by the body. Because we are removing the wastes, urine has a high nitrogen content, and can be used as a fertilizer for plants (it must be diluted with water due to the high amount of salt and nitrogen). Kidneys also actively remove some chemicals from our body, but for the most part the kidneys main role is excreting nitrogen waste, acid and salts to keep our body in balance.

# Diabetes

Our body works to keep the blood sugar (blood glucose) constant whether we are eating or not. The reason for this is that our brain cannot store sugar and needs to get it from the blood as needed. Our brain uses about one-fifth of all the energy used by our body, so the brain relies on a steady blood supply to get glucose and uses that to make the energy it uses. This means that the blood glucose level needs to keep constant, never getting too low (hypoglycemia), which would make us to pass out, or too high (hyperglycemia), and cause damage to our brain cells.

Control of the amount of sugar in the blood is done by the pancreas, an organ just below the stomach that also makes the buffers and enzymes for digestion. The pancreas makes the two hormones that control glucose: insulin and glucagon. After we eat a meal the sugar level in our blood begins to rise. The pancreas measures this and releases insulin into the blood so that liver cells will take the extra glucose and store it for later use. And then, when we have not eaten for a while and the blood glucose level starts to drop, the pancreas releases the glucagon, which makes the liver release some of that stored glucose back to the blood. This system keeps our blood glucose constant.

### Diabetes

There are medical conditions where the blood glucose levels are not controlled. If this happens for a long time, nerve cells will be damaged, especially ones that are at the ends of the body (feet, hands, but also eyes). When this happens, the high level of glucose (called hyperglycemia) causes nerve cells to die, resulting in damage to the nerves, called a neuropathy. What happens in neuropathy is that a person loses feeling on their feet or hands and begins to lose their eyesight. In losing feeling on the feet, for example, they no longer would know if they have an injury that causes pain, as pain is one of the senses that is lost. This means neuropathies lead to injury and infection, because there is no feeling in the leg or arm. If we do not feel pain when we get a cut, the infection from it can spread without us knowing.

The word used when blood glucose is not under control is diabetes mellitus. Diabetes means we are releasing a lot of water (a large urine volume) and mellitus means that it is sweet. Normally, no sugar ever gets into our urine, as we keep all of it in our body to use. But if blood sugar is not controlled, then when we eat there will be too much sugar in the blood. When blood sugar is high, some of it is dumped out by the kidneys, making the urine sweet. When this happens, we need to try and bring glucose back in balance. If we do not, many of the organs in our body can be damaged by the big changes in blood glucose. Our hormone (insulin/glucagon) regulation of blood glucose is necessary to keep normal body function. Loss of control over blood glucose leads to more damage, with neuropathies at first and later with multiple infections and then severe nerve damage (loss of sensation, loss of sight) that is life threatening.

Diabetes mellitus is first identified by having sugar in the urine (and also a larger volume of urine than usual). The first test is to measure sugar in the urine. Under normal circumstances, there is never sugar in the urine, so if there is sugar, it indicates diabetes. The two major types of diabetes mellitus are Type I, which is insulin-dependent, and Type II, which is non-insulin dependent.

### Type I Diabetes

Type I diabetes mellitus is an autoimmune disease. It usually begins during childhood, and is caused by the body's immune system destroying the part of the pancreas that makes insulin. As this happens, the person makes less and less insulin, eventually making so little that blood sugar doesn't get removed and there is too much glucose in the blood. This insulin-dependent diabetes makes big swings in the amount of glucose in the blood. The lack of insulin means that glucose does not get stored for later use, but instead stays in the blood. After eating anything, there is a sugar rush and the person feels almost dizzy with the energy rush. But several hours later, once the sugars from this meal are getting used up, the blood sugar drops below normal and the person becomes light-headed and will faint if they don't eat something. This swing in sugar is especially dangerous for the brain and nervous system, since they rely on blood sugar for all energy. If blood sugar has large changes, the nerves will get damaged. The treatment for this Type I diabetes is to closely watch blood sugar, and inject insulin each time food is eaten. There are several methods to inject insulin, by needle, a pump or an inhaler.

Type I diabetes used to mean a shortened life with many infections. But the development of injectable insulin a century ago (by Dr. William Sansum in 1922) has meant that Type I patients now have a normal life expectancy, and if they carefully watch their glucose and respond as needed they do not develop neuropathies.

### Type II Diabetes

Type II diabetes mellitus is not insulin-dependent. In Type II, the body makes plenty of insulin, but the liver cells do not respond to it. When someone has Type II diabetes, their blood sugar rises after eating, insulin gets released, and the liver does not pull the sugar out of the blood. In this case, blood glucose rises with each meal and only goes down slowly as the body uses the energy. The nervous system will also become damaged with Type II, so it must be treated.

Type II diabetes has several possible causes. Some people are at higher risk for it due to their genes, and others are at higher risk for it due to their eating patterns. The common view of how diabetes Type II starts is from frequent eating. First, we need to know that anytime we eat, this is a meal for our body. A meal can be small, like a spoon of rice, a cracker, a piece of fruit, a piece of chocolate, or tea or coffee with sugar or milk. In each of these, the carbohydrate in the snack is digested and puts sugar in the blood. The pancreas then responds by releasing insulin so that the sugar will be removed and stored. Under normal circumstances, every meal is followed by no food for hours, insulin is released, glucose levels return to normal, and insulin release stops.

In non-diabetic conditions, liver cells see insulin go up and down. They respond when there is insulin and they stop when there is no insulin. But if one meal has not been fully completed (as in digested and all the sugar stored) before the next meal starts, then the pancreas will not stop releasing insulin. In the presence of constant insulin, the liver cells no longer respond to insulin. The liver normally works by absorbing sugar when insulin is high and not absorbing sugar when insulin is low. If insulin stays elevated, the liver will gradually reset itself to treat the constant insulin level as though it is the no insulin level. When this happens, the pancreas sees that blood glucose is not decreasing, so it releases more insulin to inform the liver to absorb sugar. This increased insulin gets the liver to respond at first, but with time the liver becomes resistant to this new level of insulin in the blood and treats it as though it is the low insulin signal, and thus does not remove the sugar. This vicious circle of response to insulin becomes a big problem, and the blood sugar levels become uncontrolled.

People with higher risk for Type II diabetes are those with it in their family, and those who are overweight. If you have several relatives with Type II, you may be at higher risk. If you are obese, you are at higher risk. Some successful means to reduce risk is to reduce body weight to a normal range, to reduce or eliminate all snacks between meals (allowing only water, tea or coffee, without sugar or milk), so that there are at least four hours between each of the daily meals. Additionally, increasing physical activity is beneficial, as it helps to reduce the circulating sugar in the blood as they get used in the exercise. Eating no more than three or four times per day, reducing the total amount of food carbohydrates (so that all food has been digested by the body and put away well before the next meal) and exercising can help reduce the chances of developing Type II diabetes.

### Gestational Diabetes

Women who are pregnant have a risk of developing gestational diabetes, which is a type of diabetes that develops around the sixth month of a pregnancy. This condition affects 5 percent to 10 percent of pregnant women, and is caused by insulin resistance in the woman's body. In this case, the cause is the developing baby who needs glucose for development. The mother's pregnant body increases her blood glucose levels to give the baby the energy to grow. This can lead to a diabetic condition during the pregnancy as the insulin resistance decreases the mother's ability to control her blood glucose. The risks are for both the mother and child. The mother is at higher risk for having a Caesarean section and for developing Type II diabetes after the pregnancy (though in most cases gestational diabetes goes away after pregnancy and does not lead to Type II), and the baby is at high risk of being overweight and developing obesity and Type II diabetes as an adult.

The most successful treatment for treating or preventing gestational diabetes is to have a special meal plan and regular physical activity. Additionally, avoiding becoming overweight is very helpful, as is reducing weight if one is obese by limiting food intake and times that you eat, having a healthy diet and exercising.

# Hormones

Our body uses hormones to control many functions. Our digestion is controlled by several hormones that regulate each part of the digestive process, and then other hormones (insulin and glucagon) that keep blood sugar levels constant. Hormones are made in response to specific signals in our body and then released into our blood, and those hormones can turn on activities anywhere in the body to keep things in balance.

Hormones are released from glands, with most glands located in the head, neck or torso. The gland in the head, the pituitary, is often called the master gland because it can control many activities, including body growth, sexual function, salt balance, stress response and more.

### Thyroid-Parathyroid & Calcium

There are two glands in the neck, the thyroid gland and the parathyroid gland. These two work together to keep the calcium level in our blood steady, using our bones as a storage site for calcium. The thyroid releases calcitonin, which moves calcium from the blood to bone, while the parathyroid releases parathyroid hormone, which takes calcium out of bones and puts it back in the blood. Calcium is an important mineral in our body, and is used by all of our cells. Calcium is also necessary for bone growth and bone strength. Vitamin D is involved in this calcium cycle, as vitamin D helps us absorb calcium from our food and keeps us from losing it in our urine.

The thyroid gland has another hormone, called thyroxine,

which controls our metabolic rate. Release of this hormone is controlled by the hypothalamus in the brain, by sending a signal to the thyroid. Thyroid hormone needs iodine in our body, which is why salt is iodized (iodine is added to it). Without iodine and in some medical conditions, we may not make enough thyroxine. With low thyroxine (called hypothyroidism), an adult would have a low metabolism and can have depression and fatigue. A child with low thyroxine will have slower body and brain growth, so it is important in each case to be treated soon.

There are also conditions where the thyroid is over active (called hyperthyroidism), such as when it has a tumor or in a disease called Grave's Disease. In these cases, the growth of the thyroid gland may be seen as a goiter (a swelling in the neck region) and the person will have a high metabolic rate, may be irritable and have a fast heartbeat.

### Adrenal Gland & Cortisol

The adrenal glands sit on top of the kidneys. They have two parts, the inner part (the adrenal medulla) makes adrenaline (also called epinephrine) when we are needing to act urgently, such as when playing a soccer game or if being chased or scared. Adrenaline increases our heart and breathing and puts more glucose in the blood so we can run more.

The outer part of the adrenal gland (the adrenal cortex) makes a hormone that helps the kidney control the amount of salt in our body (aldosterone) and makes a hormone called cortisol. Cortisol release is controlled by the hypothalamus, and it has several effects. When cortisol is released into the blood for short periods of time, it speeds healing of injuries and stimulates learning. If cortisol is released into the blood for a long time (days or weeks), it has the opposite effect, slowing the healing process and stopping memories from forming.

Cortisol is released into the blood when we are stressed. If the stress is brief (an hour or part of a day), the effect is to help us divert energy to doing something to take care of the stress. But if the stress is long-term, cortisol in the blood has the effect of decreasing our digestion and immune system, increasing sugar in our blood so we can do things, and making it difficult to learn. That means the effect of stress that lasts for days or longer is to weaken our immune system and we more easily get sick.

The most effective method to reduce the effect of long-term stress on cortisol is to find ways to reduce the effect of the stress on you. Different things work for everyone, with many people finding some help from some of the following: prayer, meditation, being in nature, exercising, playing, listening to music, talking with friends, reading, etc. It is helpful to find what works for you so that you can work through stressful events.

# Reproduction

Sexual reproduction combines an egg and sperm to make one cell, called a zygote, that has half its DNA from each parent, and all its cytoplasm from the mother. This fact, that our genetic information comes half from our biological mother and half from our biological father, and that all our cell organelles come from our mother, explains why we have similar body activities as our parents. But this one fact relies on many body systems to work, from the hormonal control of reproductive function, to the development of a fetus, to childhood development and maturation. Let's go through each of these.

## *Sex Hormones*

The hypothalamus is a part of the brain, and it releases hormones that control the female and male sex hormones. When we reach puberty, the hypothalamus increases its release of gonadotropin hormone, and this gonadotropin stimulates the ovaries in women to release estrogen and progesterone and the testes in men to release testosterone. It is this increase in the sex hormones (estrogen, progesterone and testosterone) that causes the changes in a child's body so they develop as a woman or man, with the growth of breasts in women and the lowering of voice and increased body hair in men. This increase in the sex hormones also start the ability to reproduce at this age, as the ovaries start releasing an egg each month and the testes make mature sperm.

Two other hormones controlled from the hypothalamus (and

released by the pituitary, which is attached to the hypothalamus) are what controls reproduction. This means that while gonadotropin gets everything started by causing us to make more of the sex hormones, the production of eggs and sperm is controlled by these other two hormones, FSH and LH (FSH stands for follicle stimulating hormone, and LH stands for luteinizing hormone). In both women and men, FSH is what makes the eggs and sperm mature, while LH has different functions in women and men.

For the male reproductive system, sperm are produced in the testes, and this sperm production needs to be stimulated by FSH. Testosterone is also needed, and testosterone relies on LH to stimulate its release. Sperm production is pretty constant from puberty on, and begins to decrease slowly as men get older.

For the female reproductive system, FSH is released in a monthly cycle called the menstrual cycle. Menstrual cycles begin at puberty (called menarche, for first period), and end with menopause (when the hormones no longer make the menstrual cycle).

The start of a menstrual cycle is known by the day menstruation (bleeding) starts. This is called the first day of the menstrual cycle, and it is when FSH gets released, to cause an egg (called an oocyte) to mature so that it could be fertilized. Eggs in the ovaries are immature until stimulated, so that only one (or sometimes two) eggs are prepared at a time. It takes about two weeks for one egg to mature and be ready to ovulate. At this time, about fourteen days after menstruation started, an egg is mature and LH is released to cause this egg to ovulate. Ovulation means the egg leaves the ovary and travels through the oviduct to the uterus. Meanwhile, during the first half of the menstrual cycle (the first two weeks starting with menstruation), the ovaries release estrogen, which thickens the lining of the uterus called the endometrium. The endometrium is a bloody tissue that is ready for a fertilized egg. The fresh blood means that if an egg is fertilized, it can attach to the endometrium and get the nutrition it needs to grow.

Ovulation occurs in the middle of the menstrual cycle (about the fourteenth day counting from when menstruation started). If the couple has had sexual intercourse, then sperm are ejaculated into the uterus, and if an egg is present these sperm will swim toward the egg. When a couple has sexual intercourse within a few days of ovulation, they have a higher chance of becoming pregnant, because if sperm are present anywhere from five days before ovulation up to two or three days after ovulation, then the egg can be fertilized. For couples trying to get pregnant, the best odds of fertilization are to have sex the day before ovulation so the sperm are ready when the egg appears. Some women have a very regular menstrual cycle, but many do not, so this becomes difficult to predict. At ovulation, though, a woman's body temperature increases by one-half degree, and some women feel an ovulation pain from the side of their abdomen where the egg is released (it even has a name, *mittleschmertz*, from the German word for middle pain).

If an egg is fertilized by a sperm, then the second half of the menstrual cycle will have the ovary release more progesterone and estrogen. Progesterone will keep the uterus stable so the fertilized egg can attach to it and grow, and estrogen will cause more growth to occur so the uterus can grow and begin to support the developing life, and so the woman's breasts will grow to make milk for the baby. If there is no fertilization, then about two weeks after ovulation the bloody endometrium will fall off to make room for it to grow again with fresh blood.

## Pregnancy & Fetal Development

If an egg is fertilized, then a pregnancy begins. The first weeks of the pregnancy will determine if the fertilized egg, now called a zygote, will progress to a fetus. There are many factors involved, and some zygotes do not get that far, so the pregnancy ends. For the ones that do make it, over the first two months of the pregnancy, the zygote divides into many cells and begins to grow in size, becoming a fetus that is about the size of a large bean (a little more than one-half inch long). In these first two months, the growing cells get their nutrition from the endometrium, and it is the estrogen and progesterone from the ovary that keep this growing and stable. Once there's a fetus, a placenta forms around it to keep it protected. The placenta makes the estrogen and progesterone to keep the fetus growing, and the placenta connects to the fetus with the umbilical cord to provide nutrition for the fetus to grow.

The second trimester (the fourth to sixth months of the pregnancy) has a lot of development as the organs form and the brain grows and develops into its structures. The third trimester (the last three months of the pregnancy) is a time for a lot of growth of the fetus, getting it ready to be able to survive outside the womb.

In the last month of the pregnancy, the mother's hypothalamus causes the pituitary to release the hormone oxytocin, which stimulates the uterine contractions that get the baby oriented head-down to be ready to be born, and the hormone prolactin, which makes the breasts produce milk. As the day of birth gets closer, the uterine contractions happen more often, and the cervix begins to dilate (open up) so the baby's head can fit through. Once the cervix opens to 10 cm, the baby is ready to be born. The placenta breaks (the water that cushioned the fetus flows out) and the contractions get stronger until the baby's head is pushed out of the cervix and into the birth canal (the vagina) to be born.

At birth, there are fast changes for the baby, as the umbilical cord no longer carries blood and is removed, and the baby's lungs breath air for the first time.

### Early Development

With all the growth and development occurring during the pregnancy, it is important for the mother to get good nutrition and rest. Many women find that keeping active is also helpful throughout the pregnancy. Since anything the mother eats can cross over to the fetus, avoiding drugs or alcohol is important, as these can change the development of the fetus. Talk to your doctor about what to avoid, as they can help guide you through this process. It is known that exposure to alcohol, cigarette smoke, and other drugs (medical drugs, herbal drugs or recreational drugs) have an effect on the developing brain of the fetus. If possible, try to also reduce foods that may have pesticides, as the pesticides affect the nervous system and slow growth. It is best to ask your doctor about any concerns.

Once the child is born, they will mostly sleep and eat, because their brain is still growing quickly and developing after birth for the first couple of years. Their immune system also develops after birth, so it can be helpful to keep them away from anyone infectious for the first few months. After that time, it is wise to begin immunizations, to protect the child from deadly diseases. These immunizations start in the first year and continue for a few years on a schedule. Immunizations have nearly eliminated childhood death by disease, so it is important to protect your child this way.

# Development: Psychological and Social

## *Developmental Stages: Intellectual*

The intellectual development of children goes through a progression of four stages, as defined by Jean Piaget. These stages are named by the principle activity during each stage, with each stage lasting years. The stages help give some sense of why we can learn certain subjects only when we've reached a particular age level. The stages are made based on intellectual development and abilities of children at different ages, and there is agreement that each stage gives a child a more complex view of the world, that each child passes through the stages at different paces, and that no children skip a stage.

*Sensorimotor Stage*, birth to eighteen to twenty-four months. In this stage, an infant learns of the world by experiment: touching, throwing, putting objects in their mouth. In the earliest part of this stage, an infant does not have object permanence, meaning that the child does not know something exists if it is no longer seen. This is why someone can play "peek-a-boo" with a baby, covering their eyes with their hands and the baby will not appear to know why they "disappeared," being happily surprised when their hands come off and the child can see the eyes again. The development of object permanence is believed to indicate a developing memory capability. The latter part of this stage has an infant begin to use language, in a telegraphic manner (telegraphic means they just use a noun and verb, for example "go play" for I want to go and play). Babies are considered egocentric, as they do not seem to recognize that they and their parents are different people, and assume that everything is an extension of them.

*Preoperational Stage,* one and half to two years to seven years. During this stage, children begin to think symbolically, and thus are able to learn to add, subtract, multiply and divide, because numbers can represent things (this occurs at some point during this stage, for some earlier, for some later). Language becomes more advanced, with a child using sentences, and young children develop imagination and memory, and are able to differentiate between past and future. Thinking at this age is not yet fully logical, with intuition playing an important role, and their egocentricity begins to decrease.

*Concrete Operational Stage,* ages seven to eleven. These children have logical reasoning, meaning they can handle mathematics, and can also make comparisons, and can reason. They are less egocentric, beginning to realize that their thoughts are their own and not the same as others.

*Formal Operational Stage,* Age eleven and up. It is at this stage that children can think abstractly and also hypothetically. Since this is the basis for science, these children are able to use symbols to represent concepts, and can thus understand algebra and scientific analysis. They can create a hypothesis and consider it from multiple views or perspectives. They can also begin to consider and understand more abstract concepts, such as justice.

### Developmental Stages: Psycho-Social

As we develop in our personal sense of self and in our relationship to others, we go through eight broad psycho-social stages, as defined by Erik Erikson. These stages are each marked by a virtue, which plays out as a pair of contrasts, where we develop a skill or suffer the consequences of not doing so. Each of these stages identifies those who are most significant to us during this time. These stages may not be as cleanly divided as indicated here and may in fact repeat or resurface during other stages.

*Hope*, zero to two years. The key question here is "can I trust the world?" so this is a time of developing trust or learning mistrust. The most important relationship in this time is with one's mother or primary care-provider. What is happening here is a young child is learning about being cared for, and this develops into basic trust, that the world makes sense.

*Will*, two to four years. The central question at this point, "is it okay to be me?" is resolved as a child develops autonomy, or suffers shame and doubt. The central relationship is with the parents. It is during these years that a child learns some personal independence by dressing him or herelf and becoming toilet trained. This fosters the child's sense that they are okay and fit in the world around them.

*Purpose*, four to five years. This stage has family as the key relationship, and it is during this time that the child answers the question "is it okay for me to do, move and act?" In answering this, a child learns initiative, while failing to do so would have a child learn guilt. The major activities that lead to learning initiative are the child's work exploring things around them and making art.

*Competence*, five to twelve years. During these years, through the activities of school and sports, a child learns "Can I make it in the world of people and things?" The key relationships shift from family to school and neighbors, and it is during this time that a child learns to do things, or suffers from inferiority. By doing things and seeing one's own success we develop the knowledge that we can accomplish things.

*Fidelity*, thirteen to twenty years. These years are most influenced by peers and role models, and it is during this time that someone seeks to answer "who am I and who can I be?" The search for these answers allows someone to be comfortable with the identity they've chosen, while an inability to answer this leads to role confusion. Social relationships foster the process of developing answers during this period.

*Love*, twenty to forty years. This stage is when we develop intimacy, or failing that develop isolation, and the most significant relationships are with friends and partners. The question being answered during this stage is "can I love?" The means to develop the answer is through romantic relationships and other close or intimate relationships.

*Care*, forty to sixty-five years. This stage develops generativity in a person, or they have stagnation. It is the time of life when a person asks "can I make my life count?" Through this time, the significant people are from one's household and work, and it is the work itself and/or the role of parenthood that leads to the answer. These are the years one is typically highly productive at work and home, and these actions often lead to the answer.

*Wisdom*, sixty-five to death. This last stage is marked by the question "is it okay to have been me?" This stage is a reflection on one's life, where the significant relationships are with all other people, or with those you identify with. The key issue to resolve is that of having ego integrity, and those who fail this end up with despair. It is at this point in life that people reflect on their life and see all the good they have done, the love they have given and received and what they have generated, and these things provide encouragement

## Sleep and Rest

Getting sufficient sleep is essential for optimal brain function. This has become more difficult as we have greater demands placed on us, and greater access to those demands in the form of our nearly ubiquitous mobile devices. We now know that the blue spectrum of light helps stimulate us to awaken us, so reducing light in the hour before bed is helpful to allow a restful sleep. We also know that mental activity in the hour before sleep will keep our mind thinking about this in our dreams. This means that spending an hour reading before bed may continue the story in our dreams, while an hour working on a challenge may create the solution in our dreams. It also means that our minds are going to work on what we present to them, so to get sufficient rest it can be advisable to reduce strenuous mental activities in the hour before sleep. Individuals who do not get enough sleep find that they cannot think as clearly during the day, they have reduced memory, and they are prone to losing mental focus.

Time to let our brain rest in sleep is essential for both the rest of the brain, but also for setting up memories and solving challenges of the day. Just as with insufficient sleep we have difficulty remembering what we were learning, so also with sufficient sleep we are able to remember and resolve things.

## Daydreaming & Creativity

It has been shown that we take advantage of times during the day when we have no structure to daydream, and that daydreaming is a time when we have great creativity. This very activity has decreased for most people in the past decade as smart phones have become common. Now when we have a few minutes to wait, we take out our phones, while previously we daydreamed. Since the daydreaming is a creative time, our brain uses that to think up ideas or plan something. Thus, it is useful to keep unstructured times in each day that are not occupied with texts or news or games.

## *Smile*

A happy outcome from studying health and happiness is that smiling increases our appreciation of what we are experiencing, and also increases our comprehension of it. When someone's mouth is held in a smile, they are actually happier and have a positive view of what is going on around them, and when held in a frown they have the opposite response (sadder, and less aware). This means that by smiling, we can see and hear and understand better, and have a more positive outlook. Enjoy!

# Infectious Disease & the Immune System

We are surrounded by infectious microbes, all of which are too small to see. The word "microbe" means an organism that is about a micron or less in size (a micron, or micrometer, is one-thousandth of a millimeter). As we will see in the chapter on vision, the smallest things we can see are about 100 microns in size, or one tenth of a millimeter, about the thickness of one hair from our heads. Microbes include bacteria, viruses, parasites, pollen grains and yeast, among other things. And while many microbes benefit us, many others are harmful. For examples of the benefits: there are many bacteria in our digestive system that aid us with digestion; yeast (a fungus) can be used to raise bread dough or to conduct fermentation for alcohol; and pollen is used by bees to produce honey. In contrast, other kinds of bacteria can make us ill—a yeast infection can be hard to eliminate and many people suffer allergic responses to airborne pollen, while viruses can cause illness that is hard to recover from.

In fact, infections caused by bacteria and viruses used to be how most people died. In the 1800s, the average life expectancy was in the 40s, and by 1900, it was still just 47 in the US (46 for men, 48 for women). This was due to infections. In 1900, about 17% of children died in infancy in the US, while today it is about a half percent. And the life expectancy went from 47 in 1900 to 78 in 2010, an increase of 31 years (again, with women having more years than men, at 81, compared to 76 for men). This increase was partly from the lower child mortality (infant death rate), but mostly it was thanks to clean water, immunizations, and medicines like antibiotics.

While in 1900 people would wash in a bucket, reusing the same water throughout the day, now we can wash with running water. The difference is amazing! While having water to wash reduces infections, having running clean water means that everything that we wash off can no longer be in contact with us. This alone makes a huge difference in keeping infections away, for if they are washed far from us, we are no longer at risk.

By washing our hands and our food, we reduce what can get into our body. Since viruses and bacteria can survive on surfaces for hours and more, whenever we touch something and then touch our face (eye, nose or mouth), we can bring an infection into our body. This is because our skin is a fantastic barrier, not letting any infection through, but the wet surfaces of our face can allow bacteria or viruses to get into our body. Similarly, when we have a cut or sliver on our hand, this gives a path for bacteria to get under our skin, as we see when the skin turns red (from our body fighting this small infection to keep it from spreading).

So, while most of us died of infectious diseases in the 1800s, now 5% of us do, and most deaths are from chronic diseases (such as heart disease, cancer and diabetes, as explained in the other chapters in this book). Since chronic diseases are ones where we can improve things by what we eat and do, this gives us a better chance for a healthy life.

### Preventing Infections

The things that infect us are tiny, but while they are hard to see we have two important things to do to keep them from making us sick. The first is to wash with clean water. Whenever we touch anything, the bacteria and viruses that have landed there are now on our hand, and when we touch our face those microbes can enter our body through our mouth, nose or eyes. Also, if we have any open cuts in our hand, they can enter through those (they do not get through hard scabs that have formed over a cut).

Number one for preventing infections: wash our hands well. Use running water and soap (regular soap is best, antibacterial soap actually increases our risk as it gives bacteria an opportunity to evolve resistance to the antibiotic). Washing with water is always best. When water is not available, a hand sanitizer (with 60% alcohol) can help for a little while, as it works well, but is not 100% effective (sanitizer kills up to 99% of bacteria).

The second thing to do to prevent dangerous infections is to get all immunizations. While washing is important, we now also have immunizations that boost our immune system to protect us from deadly diseases such as measles, mumps, rubella, and others. If you do not have an immunization, you risk that disease harming you or your family. It was the use of water and the availability of immunizations that increased our lifespan in the past century by 30 years. Continue to do wash and get immunizations and you have the best chance of keeping healthy.

In addition to these, we know that our body fights infections best when we have a healthy diet, get regular exercise and have sufficient sleep. While there are no substitutes for these (meaning that claims of a food or herb "improving" your immune system is not true), eating healthy and exercising are things we can do and they make a difference. This book talks about food and exercise later to give ideas of how to optimize your diet and activity.

Finally, when you do get an infection, there are some medicines that can help. If it is a bacterial infection, you can get an antibiotic (antibiotics actually only work against bacteria), and if it is a viral infection, early use of an antiviral may help. These drugs only work when used at the time of infection, and we now know that taking them at other times actually weakens our response and allows the microbe to infect us.

Given all the infectious microbes around us, our bodies have a wide range of ways to stop them from entering us and making us sick. The methods our body uses come in two main categories, the general methods and the individualized ones. The general methods are often referred to as the innate defenses, or the non-specific defenses against disease, while the individualized ones are called the adaptive immune system, or the specific defenses against disease. Let's look at each of these.

### Innate Defenses

The innate defenses are good at keeping all microbes out of our body. Our first defense against infection is to keep microbes out of our body. This means our skin is first line of defense, as it is an impermeable barrier. Most infectious microbes land on the skin and have no way through. And the skin also has secretions of oil and sweat that keep the skin healthy and also inhibit microbial growth. The only way through the skin is when we have a cut. And once we do have a hole in our skin, we immediately have bacteria invading. Indeed, this is why your skin gets red when you have a sliver or a small cut: the bacteria on that sliver have now entered the body and have started the local action called inflammation that isolates them and gets rid of them.

This means the main way we keep microbes out is the lining of our body, with its various secretions. This includes the skin with its acidic sweat, which slows bacterial growth, and its antimicrobial secretions that damage bacteria as well as activate action under the skin. Other skin-like linings include the openings in our body, each of which has its own secretions. Our ears and the waxy secretion that protects the eardrum; our airways with the mucus that traps dust entering and cilia that move that material back out; our mouth that feeds into the stomach where the strong acid destroys most microbes; the urethra that has acidic urine flowing out and keeps bacteria from growing, and the vagina which also is acidic to inhibit bacterial growth. Our eyes are also protected, producing tears to lubricate and making an enzyme called lysozyme that breaks apart bacterial walls to destroy them.

Each of these methods is essentially a fortified barrier. The barrier is the lining that keeps microbes from getting to cells that could be infected and the fortification is the secretions that inhibit bacteria and can break them apart.

Once inside the body, however, there are other important innate protections against infection. One of these is fever. When we have a bacterial infection, there are white blood cells that recognize the bacteria and send an alarm by releasing a signaling chemical into the blood. This chemical is called a pyrogen (fire generator). It travels in the blood vessels and stimulates cells in the hypothalamus of the brain that regulate body temperature. When pyrogen is present, our body temperature rises. We often feel this as sweat and chill. The reason we feel these apparent changes in body temperature is due to the temperature control point and the actual body temperature, much like raising the temperature in a home, where we adjust the setting and then the heat turns on. When the brain sees pyrogen, the set point for our body temperature is raised, but it takes time for us to heat up. For this time, we feel very cold, which of course drives us to put on warmer clothes. And then, because the higher set point is not as stable as our normal temperature, we may pass it, or the pyrogen level may fluctuate, and we then feel very hot and try to cool back down. This gives us the sense of having fever and chills.

Another important innate protection is inflammation. Inflammation occurs when foreign microbes get exposed to our blood. When they do, a type of white blood cell (called a mast cell) recognizes the foreign microbe and releases a chemical signal to protect the body. This chemical is histamine. Histamine makes blood capillaries in the area expand (dilate), bringing more blood into the infected region, and it makes these capillaries leakier so that the protective white blood cells can seek out and destroy the microbes that have entered the body. This increased blood flow creates most of the four signs of inflammation: redness, swelling, warmth and pain. The increased blood flowing into the infected area is warm and red and it swells that area. The pain is due to the tissue damage and the microbes activating pain receptors, so that we are quickly aware of the injury. You likely have observed that when you cut your hand or have a splinter you feel pain, and the area becomes warmer, redder and swollen. This is the inflammatory response, part of our innate immune system.

Some of the white blood cells that enters the area are phagocytes. A phagocyte is a white blood cell (cyte) that eats (phago) foreign cells and debris. These white blood cells recognize the foreign microbes and swallow them and break them apart. In this way the bacteria are destroyed and unable to infect our body outside of the local area where they first arrived.

### Recognizing Foreign Microbes

How do phagocytes know something is foreign? They can recognize the unique code that is on the surface of almost all cells. This code is called the major histocompatibility complex (MHC). The MHC is a unique identifier on nearly every cell in our body. The MHC is identical for all the cells in one body, but is different from the cells in another body. This means that each person, each animal, every living thing has an identifying marker on the surface of each cell to indicate whether a cell is "self" or "not-self." If it is self, we let it be, if it is not-self, we can have a phagocyte eliminate it.

Some fascinating aspects of these cell markers are that when one of our cells becomes infected with a virus, the virus places its code on the surface, which will allow our body to recognize it as infected. Additionally, the MHC surface marker is likely a problem in autoimmune conditions, where the body targets and destroys cells in itself that are necessary for normal function (as is the case for diabetes Type I). It may be that the cell surface is modified such that the body sees it as foreign instead of a self cell.

It is also these cell surface markers that make organ transplantation so challenging. Once the donor organ is in the patient, the patient's defense system will try to destroy this foreign material. For this reason, even though the donor and recipient are matched by blood type and such, organ transplant recipients need to take drugs that suppress their immune system so the transplanted organ will continue to function without being damaged by the body's defenses. Additionally, when blood is to be transfused, this is why the blood types are matched and then cross-matched (tested) to minimize the risk of a reaction against the donor blood.

### Adaptive Immunity

When infectious microbes get past our innate immunity, then they have entered our body and have access to our blood vessels. But once they have access to the blood, the blood also has a route to follow to get to the infection. This is when our adaptive immune system gets into action. The adaptive immune system relies on specialized cells that recognize not only that something is foreign, but exactly which type of infection it is. In much the same way that we have cell surface markers to indicate self and not-self, there are additional markers on the cell surface that indicate what particular organism it is. These markers can identify if a bacterium is a beneficial one that makes yogurt or a dangerous one that creates a staph infection. Each different organism has a marker on its surface, and our adaptive immune cells are able to recognize many millions of different markers.

There are two types of adaptive immune cells. Both of these cell types are lymphocytes, meaning they live in lymph tissue. Recall that the lymphatic system, which we discussed in the blood vessel section of the heart chapter, are low pressure, fluid-filled vessels that return fluid from the periphery of our body to the heart and circulatory system. The lymphatic system has a one way flow due to valves inside it, and it has a series of lymph nodes that the fluid passes through. The nodes have a critical function: this is where the lymphocytes reside and as the fluid goes past the lymphocytes, they can see what is in it. If we have an infection, the lymphocytes in the nearest lymph node will be the first to find out.

The two classes of lymphocytes in the adaptive immune system are the B cells and the T cells. They earned these names based on the locations there were originally found (bursa of Fabricius for B cells and thymus for T cells). In humans, these B and T cells are formed in the bone marrow (B cells) and thymus and tonsils (T cells), following which they mostly migrate to the lymph nodes and stay there through our life.

When there is a foreign cell in our body, as it travels through the lymph node it is recognized, and the B cells and T cells begin the process to destroy the foreign microbe.

Each class of lymphocyte is best for different infections. B cells are optimal for attacking bacteria and T cells for destroying virally infected cells. Both types of lymphocytes are essential to our defense against disease.

## B Cells & Antibodies

Once a B cell recognizes a specific microbe, it makes two groups of B cells, one that makes antibodies and the other that remembers the infection. Antibodies are large proteins that grab a marker on the infecting microbe. Antibodies travel around in the blood, reaching all areas of the body. When they find a marker they can bind (called the antigen), they stick to it. By binding on an antigen, the antibody stops infectious bacteria from working, and more significantly, the antibody puts a label on the infectious microbe that is used by macrophages (white blood cells that phagocytize foreign cells) to quickly grab it and break it up.

The B cells that remember the infection stay in the lymph node. Their only job is to remember this antigen. When we are infected by the same infection again, these memory B cells quickly convert to making antibody. While the first time we are exposed to a disease, it takes days to produce enough antibody to fight the infection (which is why we feel sick for a couple days), when we are exposed again, the antibody production is immediate, resulting in us not getting sick at all.

## T Cells & Killer Cells

T cells are activated similarly, with the T cell making groups of cytotoxic cells, also known as killer cells, memory cells and helper cells. Unlike B cells, the killer T cells leave the lymph node and travel in the blood to find the infected cells. Once the killer T cells find an infected cell, they hold onto it and break its membrane to destroy the cell by making a hole in the infected cell, which allows water to go in and break the cell apart. Phagocytes then come into the area to clean up the debris.

Because killer T cells destroy infected cells, they are our main protection from viruses. When a virus enters our body, it needs to go inside our cells in order to have the equipment to make more viruses. It takes over our own body cell to make more viruses, which then travel out to other body cells and infect more. Killer T cells recognize the infected cells that are in our body and deliberately destroy them to stop the infection.

Memory T cells stay in the lymph node to remember the antigen. When we get the same virus, we quickly make killer T cells, which find the infected cells and destroy them before we feel ill. Again, the first infection is felt because it takes days to make enough killer T cells the first time. Once we have memory cells, they quickly make killer T cells and fight the infection the first day, knocking it out before we feel it.

### Immunizations

This ability for memory B and T cells to remember an infection is how immunizations work. Diseases that used to spread to millions each year now are kept down by each of us getting an immunization. These shots work by giving us an inactive form of the microbe, so our immune system makes memory cells. When we do get exposed, we are "immune" from the infection because our immune system attacks it before it harms us.

If the memory cells remember the viral infection, then why do they not fight the flu (influenza virus) each time? This is because there are many variations of the flu virus. Each year one strain afflicts millions of people. But the next year it is a different strain. We can become sick from the flu each year because it is a different flu virus each time.

One new type of treatment for cancer is to take killer cells from a person's blood, grow them in culture to produce more copies of these same cells, and modify them to recognize a cancer that is in the person's body. When these cells are put back into the body, the results have been very promising in terms of destroying much of the cancer with the power of our own body.

## Cytokines and AIDS

The helper T cells have a different job. They make signals called cytokines. These cytokines are made when we are infected, and they boost the immune response of both the B and T cell systems, as well as enhance the activity of the phagocytes. Cytokines are our immune enhancers. It is important that they only increase when we have an infection. In studies where they were artificially increased for a longer time, it was found that the boost from the cytokines only lasts for days, after which the immune system stops responding to them.

A reason we know about cytokines is that in acquired immunodeficiency syndrome (AIDS), the virus HIV (human immunodeficiency virus) kills helper T cells. With time, these infected helper T cells no longer produce the cytokines we need, and we are no longer able to fight infections. In this way, a cold can become deadly, as the body is unable to fight it off.

## Boosting the Immune System

The immune system does an impressive job of fighting off infections. As we age, the number of lymphocytes and their effectiveness decreases, so an infection that may have made us sick for one day when we were twenty may last a few days at seventy. The things we can do to help our immune system perform at its peak involve having a healthy diet (high in fruits and vegetables), get regular exercise (walking forty-five minutes a day), do not smoke or vape, keep a healthy weight, get enough sleep, and reduce stress. As is talked about in the nervous system chapter, stress hurts our digestive and immune systems by sapping energy from them and diverting it to use on stress. When the immune system gets less energy, it cannot operate optimally, and we get sick. This is why students often get sick after final exams. They have been working hard, losing sleep and being stressed. This works to weaken their immune system and they more quickly get a cold. Reducing stress and getting enough sleep are essential for a healthy immune system. Other things to do are drink alcohol only in moderation (if you drink), wash your hands often, and fully cook any meats you eat.

# Nervous System

The human brain is made of almost 100 billion neurons, with current estimates at approximately 86 billion. It also has an equal number of glial cells, which are the cells that support neurons. But it is not simply the number of neurons or the physical size of a brain that give us abilities. We think intelligence is related to the location of these neurons in the different areas of the brain, and how many connections they make.

## Neurons and Glial Cells

The cells that make up the nervous system are neurons and glial cells. Neurons are able to conduct electrical impulses along their length through a long extension of the cell called an axon. Axons are very thin and long tubular extensions of a neuron. They carry electrical impulses along their length to terminal endings, where the electrical impulses release small chemical signals, called neurotransmitters. These neurotransmitters communicate between one neuron and the next. This chemical communication between two neurons is called a synapse. All neurons have synapses, and most of them have many thousands of synapses to other neurons. At these synapses, the information sent as chemical neurotransmitters is processed and because of this processing, each synapse is similar to a simple computer circuit, processing the impulses being sent. Since the impulses are on/off signals, they act like a binary system, which communicates with 1s and 0s.

In addition to neurons, we have an approximately equal number of glial cells in our nervous system. These glial cells have a wide variety of support activities, from taking care of the environment around neurons and helping produce certain molecules, to wrapping around axons to insulate them and speed up the impulses by a hundred fold. This wrapping is called myelin, and since the glial cell wrapping is primarily made of cell membrane, it is an oily substance that reflects light to make the axons look white. In contrast, the cell bodies have no coating and are gray. Since it is near the cell bodies where the information processing synapses are located, when someone says they are using their "gray matter," this is an expression for saying they are thinking.

Because neurons are very active and have no means to store energy, they need a constant blood supply to provide their nutrients. It is estimated that our brain receives about one fifth of the blood supply for our body, and that it needs this supply all the time. To help give good access to the blood, the cell bodies of neurons are located near the surface of the brain, where the blood capillaries are concentrated. This means that the top few millimeters of the brain surface are primarily cell bodies, and the myelin-coated axons connect the regions.

One think about brain surface is that the brain is very folded. If you see a brain, it looks all wrinkled from the folding, making brain surface almost everywhere inside the skull. As our brain develops, it folds in and over on itself many times. This increases the surface area that fits inside the skull. Since cell bodies are near the surface, that means human brains have maximized the numbers of neurons that can be packed into the skull by folding the surface of the brain repeatedly.

This folding is a common feature in human structures; we fold the surfaces of organs that need a large area to exchange nutrients while minimizing the total volume. Perhaps the most extreme example is our lungs, which have over 100 square meters (over 1,000 square feet) of surface area packed into our upper chest! Since lungs need to absorb enough oxygen from the air to support our entire body, they do this by maximizing surface area in a minimal volume. Our brains take advantage of this same concept to facilitate getting oxygen into the cells.

### Central and Peripheral Nervous System

Our nervous system has several clear regions. There is the central nervous system, made of the brain and spinal cord, and the peripheral nervous system made up of all the nerves outside of the brain and spinal cord. The peripheral system is responsible for taking in sensory information about the world around us, as well as sending out the messages to do things like talk or walk.

The central nervous system is arranged into spinal cord, hindbrain, midbrain and forebrain. These four sections each have their major functions. The spinal cord is responsible for transmitting information (sensory and movement) to the appropriate area and for providing reflexes. The hindbrain regulates the essential and subconscious body functions of breathing, digestion, cardiovascular, etc. The midbrain handles auditory and visual reflexes that let us walk without hitting things. The forebrain is the largest part of our brain; it processes all sensory and movement information, is the area of conscious control and decision making, and is the region that provides both volition and reasoning.

Within the hindbrain are the brainstem and the cerebellum. The brainstem is the part of the brain that keeps a body alive, controlling the breathing and heart, along with digestion. The cerebellum is behind the brainstem. It has the role of coordinating all movements, to fine tune the plan for each movement with the sensory information of how the movement is proceeding. It is the cerebellum that makes our movements smooth, by using constant feedback about how the movement is proceeding to make it both well-planned and well-executed. The cerebellum has perhaps the densest array of neurons in the brain, with more than half of the neurons in this one structure working to smooth our movements and help us keep balanced. It is because of this structure that we can walk on a balance beam smoothly, write our name consistently, and speak articulately. When our cerebellum is temporarily impaired, as when someone consumes alcohol, this smoothness of our movements is lost and we stumble as we walk, write poorly, and slur our speech. The effect of many other drugs on the cerebellum is similar to alcohol. When any of these are combined with sleep deprivation, the mis-function is magnified.

## Autonomic Nervous System

A large part of the peripheral nervous system is what has been given the name autonomic nervous system. This is not a separate system, it is the part of the peripheral system that increases and decreases groups of body systems. Autonomic nerves send the information to increase and decrease the heart or respiration, for example, which is  determined by the brain's measure of the oxygen and carbon dioxide in our blood. The autonomic system has two divisions: sympathetic and parasympathetic. The sympathetic is the branch that increases breathing and heart rate, while the parasympathetic decreases these. When we eat a meal, the parasympathetic increases digestion and builds up the immune system. These two divisions work together, with the sympathetic division increasing our physical activity, increasing our adrenalin when we are excited, and letting us use move quickly to escape a situation. The parasympathetic division restores energy in the body and helps us get our needed rest. When one system is active, the other one is inactive. For example, when you run to catch a train, your sympathetic system is activated, but when you sit to eat a meal, your parasympathetic system is active.

### Stress and Illness

When our parasympathetic nerves are active, we strengthen our immune system. When our sympathetic nerves are active, we take energy from everywhere to use to move. Since the sympathetic system is activated by stress, when we have prolonged stress that lasts for more than a few days, we weaken our immune system and more easily get sick. This is why someone caring for a partner who is sick will get more illnesses him or herself.

### Cerebral Cortex-the Large Part of our Brain

The largest part of our brain is the two hemispheres of cerebrum, which are usually referred to as the cerebral cortex. The word cortex means outer part of an organ, while medulla means the inner part of an organ. In the brain, the cortex, or surface, of the brain is very folded. Because there are two hemispheres, we refer to them as the right and the left hemisphere. The hemispheres have four distinct lobes, the frontal, parietal, occipital and temporal lobes. Each lobe has a primary responsibility. The temporal lobes, which are on the sides of the brain and between our eyes and ears, process sound, and it is in this lobe that we understand language, translating the sounds into concepts. For individuals who speak words in multiple languages, the language comprehension area is larger. It is also believed that this area may allow us to hear music as something more like a language, where ideas are communicated, than a series of notes.

The occipital lobes, which are at the very back of the head, processes visual information, taking the information from the eyes and making sense of it. The parietal lobes are at the top of the brain, and these receive all the sensory information from our body, indicating how we are moving, what is touching us, the temperature on our skin and so on.

The frontal lobes are in the front of the brain, just behind our forehead. These lobes create all movements of our body. Since language is a complex coordinated movement, the frontal lobes are the part of the brain that speaks. The frontal lobes are also the place where we make decisions, think, create ideas, and have our personality. When we understand that the frontal lobes are responsible for all movements, we begin to see our personality as movements: the movement of our arms and face, the way we speak, and so on.

Near the very center of the brain, and under all the lobes, is a structure called the thalamus. The thalamus is a relay center for almost all of our sensory information. Each sense first sends the information to the thalamus, and the thalamus sends it on to the specific lobe that processes that information. Surrounding the thalamus are a series of smaller structures that are important for smell, learning, emotion, and maintenance of our body's internal conditions. Because these parts are close together, they affect each other. For example, many smells have emotional impacts on us. Also, events that are very emotional increase our memory of them.

### Homeostasis-Keeping Things in Balance

The part of our brain that controls our body's internal environment is just below the thalamus, and is called the hypothalamus. This small brain part is responsible both for our circadian rhythms and for our homeostasis. Homeostasis means body constancy, and it refers to the fact that we keep our body's internal environment (temperature, fluid levels, etc.) constant despite the constant changes around us. This constancy allows us to not be influenced by outside conditions such as cold or heat. The hypothalamus does this by making a set point, and then continually monitoring and adjusting to keep conditions at the set point. The hypothalamus does this by changing our behavior and our hormones. Since the hypothalamus is part of the brain, it sends signals the change our behavior, such as being thirsty when our fluids are low so we drink water. The hypothalamus is also directly connected to the pituitary gland, which secretes hormones that stimulate the growth spurts of our body, control water balance and blood pressure, regulate our reproductive systems and fertility, control the thyroid gland (which regulates metabolism), and establish the conditions for pregnancy and childbirth. One example of how the hypothalamus works is seen by considering body temperature, which is kept at a constant 37C (98.6F). When it is cold around us, we have the behavior "I'm cold" and put on warmer clothes as well as increase our metabolism and shiver, all of which increase heat in our body. When it is hot, we have the opposite behavior, and we remove coats, and even sweat, to remove heat.

### Lateralization-the Difference between Left and Right

The brain is lateralized, meaning that some functions are located more on one side than the other. This is true for language, which is primarily on the left side of the brain for most people (both language comprehension and speaking). This is believed to be true for nearly all right-handed people and to be true for half or more of left-handed people. There are other lateralized brain functions, although it is not noticeable since we have a rapid communication between the two halves of the brain so each side knows everything happening in both sides of the brain. In general, there seems to be more calculation type thinking on the left side of the brain and more spatial thinking on the right side. This has given rise to the notion that the left side is the mathematical side and the right side is the artistic side.

Another lateralization is that all the information coming from the left side of the body crosses over and goes to the right side of the brain, and vice versa. Similarly, the right side of the brain moves the left side of the body, so this crossing occurs both for incoming and outgoing signals. The only exception to this is the sense of smell, which does not cross over.

## Neurotransmitters-the Brain's Signaling Molecules

The synapses between neurons are how we process and store information. These synapses are individually very small but, as mentioned above, we have a huge number of them. We also add new synapses as we learn. The method of communication at each synapse is to use a signaling molecule called a neurotransmitter. There are a chemicals used by the body as neurotransmitters. All of them are small molecules, and all of them work similarly. The difference is that each chemical has different effects on the receiving cell. The more common chemicals used as neurotransmitters are:

| Neurotransmitter | Major Actions |
|---|---|
| Acetylcholine | Movement; Memory |
| GABA | Most common inhibitory signal |
| Glutamate | Most common excitatory signal |
| Dopamine | Movement; Reward |
| Serotonin | Mood; Arousal |
| Norepinephrine | Arousal; Mood |

The action of a neurotransmitter depends on the chemical used and the cells that are receiving it. The two most common neurotransmitters are glutamate and GABA. Glutamate is used in about one quarter of all brain synapses. It can do things like communicate information about vision or create new memories. And since it is so common, if someone is particularly sensitive to excess glutamate in their diet it can result in headaches. This is the case for a number of people when they eat the spice MSG (monosodium glutamate). This spice stimulates two flavors on our tongue: saltiness and umami, or meatiness. It is the glutamate in MSG that provides the umami taste, and for some people, added MSG can increase glutamate in the blood and then get to some areas and cause a headache. The most effective solution to avoid the headaches if you are sensitive to MSG is to reduce or eliminate this spice.

## Pharmacology-Why Drugs Affect Us

Because each of our synapses uses a chemical neurotransmitter, if we take a drug that acts like this transmitter, we can mimic the effect of it. Similarly, if we take a drug that blocks the transmitter, we can reduce or even stop its effect. We call the mimic drugs agonists, and the blocking drugs antagonists. The study of how such drugs work is pharmacology. Since these drugs affect neurotransmitters in our brain, they can change our mental state or our perceptions or behavior.

Using some drugs can be beneficial for several neurological conditions, especially if used at similar levels to what is naturally in the brain. However, if higher amounts of the drug are used, the brain cells can desensitize to it, requiring even higher amounts for an effect. Also, some drugs can be used to create an altered mental state. While these drugs are acting on normal brain functions, they often are at substantially higher levels than our brain uses, and this can create side effects when we take the drug at high levels. For example, morphine is a drug that acts on the opioid pathways in the brain. These pathways reduce our feeling of pain, and so morphine is used to reduce severe pain. The challenge is that when the opioid pathway is stimulated at higher levels, it creates a need for regular stimulation (called dependency). Also, there is a side effect of opioids in that they suppress breathing at very high doses. If someone abuses morphine or any opioid drug, and adapts to its presence so that they need to use higher amounts of it, they can reach a point where they stop breathing. When this happens, they need immediate medication that stops the opioid effect so that they will continue to breathe. The current opioid drug addiction problem in the United States shows just how strongly addictive these narcotics are, as people who were prescribed them for pain kept using them after the pain was gone because of the dependency the opioids caused. As they continued to use the drugs, they desensitized and used greater amounts, which has resulted in many deaths and emergency calls.

## Pharmacology-Some Drugs that Affect the Brain

There are many drugs used that affect our nervous system, with opioids being one. The drugs that affect the brain include ones that increase production of a neurotransmitter, such as using L-DOPA to help neurons make the dopamine they are lacking in Parkinson's disease, or the antipsychotic medications that reduce dopamine in order to treat schizophrenia. Other treatments use an SSRI (selective serotonin reputake inhibitor) such as fluoxetine or St. John's Wort to restore serotonin levels in some cases of depression, or using marijuana to treat the severe nausea from cancer or multiple sclerosis and help patients regain their energy by being able to eat. Marijuana itself has a number of compounds that affect us, including stopping nausea, but also including putting us into an altered state and interfering with memory and brain development, which is why it is not often prescribed for those under twenty-five, as it has long-term effects on their brain development if used regularly.

# Brain and Nerve Disorders

## Parkinson's Disease

In Parkinson's disease, a particular part of the brain is not able to make enough of the neurotransmitter dopamine, resulting in a person having weaker control of their movement. This is seen as a tremor (shaking) in the hands, and slurred speech, both of which progress so that the whole body may shake and eventually a person may be unable to move. Since the problem is not enough dopamine, by giving the person a precursor for dopamine, L-DOPA, their neurons are able to make dopamine again for a while, and this eases the problem. With time, they adapt to this added compound. One of the solutions that provide help later is called deep brain stimulation. This involves surgically implanting an electrode in the region of the brain where the problem is to stimulate it directly. Doing this gets around the need to use a drug that the brain can adapt to, which gives hope for a longer-term solution.

## Stroke

A stroke is a loss of blood flow to a part of the brain. The loss can happen because of a blockage in a blood vessel, which is called an ischemic stroke. The loss can happen instead because of a ruptured blood vessel in the brain, and this is called a hemorrhagic stroke. About two-thirds of strokes are ischemic, and one third hemorrhagic. When a stroke happens, the loss of blood flow means that neurons are starved for oxygen and cannot make energy. When they lose energy for hours, these cells will die, and with them is the loss of a specific activity. Because it takes a few hours for the cells to die, ischemic strokes can be treated medically by giving a patient a drug that dissolves blood clots, or by removing the clot. This is done in a hospital setting, and can result in little damage for the person if treated quickly. Hemorrhagic strokes are not treatable in this manner, but can be operated on to stop the leaking blood. This is a much more delicate procedure. As a result, while most strokes are ischemic, more of the deaths are from hemorrhagic strokes. Ischemic strokes have a death rate of about 40 percent, while hemorrhagic strokes are close to 90 percent. The most important factor in survival of a stroke is how quickly someone has medical attention. The next factor is receiving therapy to relearn the skills that were damaged by the stroke.

If you see someone who suddenly has slurred speech, or is not able to move an arm or leg, immediately call 911. Your quick action will be essential for their condition.

The chief risk factor for stroke is high blood pressure, with other risks including high cholesterol levels, obesity, diabetes, smoking and atrial fibrillation. Strokes are a disease that increase with age, with two-thirds of all strokes occurring in those over sixty-five years of age. Treatments to reduce the likelihood of a stroke include having a healthy diet and getting regular exercise, along with medication that reduces clot formation for those at higher risk.

### Depression, Phobias, OCD & Schizophrenia

It is estimated that more than one out of ten people in the US have a mood disorder in any given year, so these are very common, and they are treatable. There are a number of mood disorders, including clinical depression, fears (called phobias), obsessive-compulsive disorder (OCD), bipolar disorder and schizophrenia. In each of these diseases, there are several treatment options. For the first three listed, therapy is often the best treatment with or without some medication, while bipolar disorder and schizophrenia typically require medication plus therapy. Therapy has been shown to help a person understand what is causing their condition and learn how they can handle it by thinking of different ways to view things. This coping strategy often benefits the person, who learns that they have the power to make a difference. When therapy alone is insufficient, there are a number of drugs that can be used in combination with therapy, with a common type of drug for depression being an SSRI (selective serotonin reuptake inhibitor). These drugs work to increase the levels of serotonin in certain areas of the brain, and are often helpful in treating mood disorders because natural serotonin levels are usually lower in these diseases. There are several pharmacological versions of the SSRI drugs, and also at least one herbal version (St. John's Wort). Because they work the same way, do not use both at the same time as it is dangerous for you. Lithium has also been used for mood disorders, and seems to work to increase serotonin levels in a different way than an SSRI does. Lithium is a mineral that our body can absorb, but does not get rid of very quickly, so taking too much of it is also harmful. Some mood disorders may be due to a vitamin deficiency in the brain.

Depression (also called unipolar depression) is often triggered by some event, and a person dwells on its effect, making it very difficult to do anything. Depression has been increasing among young people, often due to stress. It is always best to talk to your medical person about it to get the support needed to treat depression because if not treated it will often come back later. Phobias are common among children, with about one in four children having fears that can develop into a phobia. While many children outgrow their fear, others develop a phobia from it. It is wise to allow a child to talk about their fear and to treat what they say with respect.

Guidance from a medical professional will help. OCD also seems to have its roots in adolescence, when we are learning to make structure in our life. For this, too, talk with your medical professional. Again, showing respect for the child describing this is helpful.

Bipolar disorder causes people to alternate between depression and mania. Mania is a wildly enthusiastic state. Medication helps even out these swings and allows a person to do well. Schizophrenia is a psychotic disorder that affects about one in a hundred people and usually develops when someone is in their twenties. It causes hallucinations and also a low emotional state and is treated with antipsychotic medication.

An excellent source of information on mental health disorders is the NIH (National Institutes of Health) site that details many conditions and provides current understanding about each of them: http://nimh.nih.gov/health/

### Autism Spectrum Disorder (ASD)

Autism spectrum disorder (ASD) is the name given to a range of conditions where a person has difficulty with social interactions. The previous name for some of these was Asperger Syndrome. These individuals typically have trouble identifying emotions and facial expressions in other people, have challenges in understanding someone else's point of view, and difficulty in communicating because of this. ASD usually develops in childhood and is thought to be more common in males. These children often are good at learning things, especially in the sciences and arts. These individuals often do better with a daily routine, as changes are difficult for them, and therapy can be helpful for them to understand and develop coping methods. Some studies have indicated that people with ASD may have less recognition of faces, meaning that they not only may not recognize expressions, they may not be able to recognize the face of someone. We know that there is a facial recognition part of our brain (in the right hemisphere) that allows us to see faces. This is such a strong feature that we frequently see faces where there is none, such as on mountains or clouds or other inanimate objects. It may be that an aspect of ASD is to affect this part of the brain.

The number of children diagnosed with ASD has been increasing and has doubled in the past decade to about 2%. Recent studies show that certain foods may be affecting some children in a way that increases their difficulty in communication. Given the preference of ASD children for the same food each day, it would be hard to make a change, but having them help in preparing food and involving them in reducing meat and dairy may be helpful.

## Eating Disorders

There are a range of eating disorders, from not eating enough to eating too much. The part of the brain that controls our eating is in the hypothalamus. It is here that we respond to needing nutrition or energy by feeling hungry, and it is also here that we know we have eaten enough by feeling sated. The hypothalamus also maintains our circadian clock, so our hunger is often synchronized with our mealtimes. The frequency of eating disorders has increased in recent decades, and the reasons are still unclear. All eating disorders result in physical problems, so it is important to address them. Eating disorders often begin during the teenage years, but can start at any age, and are more common in women. They seem to be affected by, or coexist with other conditions such as OCD, or depression, or socializing issues. The individuals also tend to be smart, and this leads to more successful treatment plans, which are to help the person want to address the problem and come up with a solution. Because the disorder retrains the hypothalamus, when the individual afflicted is able to address the disorder, they are more successful at training themselves to recognize the hunger and satiety signals their brain puts out.

## Post Traumatic Stress Disorder (PTSD)

PTSD is a condition that arises in some people who undergo a dangerous or frightening event. The condition usually develops within months of the trauma, and it is estimated that it afflicts over 5 percent of people at some point in their life, with women being at higher risk for it than men. While it often follows trauma, it may also occur in someone who loses a loved one or who has a loved one that experiences trauma. It is difficult to treat, with the most common methods being medications and therapy. A helpful therapy is cognitive behavioral therapy (CBT), which helps people face and control their fear and to revise how they think of the trauma-causing event (usually by addressing any guilt or shame they feel and help them recognize it is not their fault).

## Stress

Stress is a challenge to the nervous system that uses body resources to respond to the stress event. Short term stress results in a rush of adrenalin and an increase in cortisol, both of which increase blood sugar to increase movement, speed up heart and lung rates to deliver energy to the body faster, and enhance learning for a short time so we learn how to respond better to the challenging situation next time. Examples of short-term stress can include being in danger or in a competition. In either situation, the stressor lasts a short time (minutes to hours), the body responds with a burst of activity to react quickly, and we remember the event to allow us to respond more quickly the next time.

In contrast, long-term stress (stress lasting many days or weeks) activates the same systems, but the longer duration of this increase in energy delivered in the body serves to reduce rest, suppress learning and minimize creative thinking (making it difficult to identify solutions to the stress). Thus, the rush of adrenalin and cortisol that increased problem solving and action in the short-term situation harm these same actions when the stress is long-term. Examples of long-term stress include caring for an ill loved one or devoting a large amount of time to a project or school. In these cases, body energy is drained by nervous activity, creativity is stifled, and learning is impaired. We know from brain studies that the learning area of the brain decreases in synaptic contacts with long-term stress (as well as with PTSD).

Solutions for stress are to eliminate or reduce the stressor, engage in stress-reducing activities (these vary by person, with some solutions being physical activity, some relaxation, some prayer or meditative, some conversing and laughing), eat a healthy diet and get enough sleep. Since stressors tend to reduce these activities, it requires more work to do them when we are stressed, but doing so can help reduce the difficulties brought on by the stress response.

### Dementia

There are many types of dementia, and most of them arise later in life. The most well-known dementia is Alzheimer's, which is characterized by a buildup of some proteins in the brain. Alzheimer's has several signs, particularly being unable to remember plans, and an increasing loss of memories. Confusion is common, and as the disease progresses a patient may not know that they don't know.

Senile dementia, which means age-related dementia, is characterized by a loss of memory for specific events, which also gradually increases. Senile dementia patients often seem to know that they cannot remember something, and this makes them frustrated or angry. In these people, there is often "sundowning," which refers to how late in the afternoon they seem to have reached their limit of trying to think and remember for the day; they display more frustration with things around them and may speak out as though they are angry.

Research is trying to find solutions to treat dementia of all types. So far, we have learned that diet and activity are important, as is mental activity. Having a healthy cardiovascular system may give someone an advantage in getting oxygen to the brain and slow development of dementia. Having a rounded diet with high levels of vitamins and low levels of saturated fats and salt seem to be helpful. It is best not to smoke, perhaps because smoking decreases oxygen in the brain. Moderate exercise may be helpful because it improves the cardiovascular system, and mental exercises (solving puzzles or problems, reading, thinking) seem to be helpful as well.

## Language Disorders

In the first year of life, all of us have the capacity to learn any language. We can make every sound of every language at that time, and over the first year we only continue making the sounds that we hear. This means that the way we learn language is by hearing it and mimicking it. Over the next two decades of our life, we acquire words and grammar at a phenomenal pace, greatly increasing our capacity in our native languages. Additionally, other languages that are learned at an early age typically are learned with fluency. In this way, someone who learns a language in the first years of life speaks the same as a native speaker, with no accent. It is when we learn a language later in life that we often learn it with our native language accent more pronounced. This is in large part because as we develop familiarity with the languages of our youth, we lose the ability to distinguish sounds that are not part of the languages we speak. If we cannot hear the difference, we cannot reproduce the difference, and we have a limit in our language skill. This does not affect learning languages that are similar to our native language, but it makes learning a language that is much different from ours a lot more difficult.

The ability to accurately hear a language is critical in learning language in the first years of life. If a child has recurrent ear infections (ear infections that occur one after another), their hearing is clouded by the fluid buildup in the ear, and this fluid muffles the sounds they hear. If the ear infections do not clear up, the child will very accurately reproduce these muffled sounds as they learn their language. In this case, once the child begins speaking, it will be obvious that they are not speaking correctly. The first assumption is often that there is an impediment (a difficulty) in their ability to speak, but the impediment is usually in their ability to hear. Once the ear infections are cleared, the child can hear and make the correct sounds. If ear infections are frequent in the first two to three years, a child can have difficulty reproducing language correctly.

## *Motivation*

Motivation is viewed as a hierarchy of needs, with the ultimate goal of being a self-actualizing, creative person. To accomplish this, we understand that some needs must be met before we can handle others. The most basic needs are survival ones, such as air, food and water. Once basic needs are met, then safety needs can be addressed. Safety needs include housing, security of employment and personal safety. Those who have met the safety needs can then try to satisfy the need to love and be loved (to belong). The love need includes family, friends and intimate partners, and is how we feel we belong somewhere. Those who have met the love needs can begin to address esteem needs. Esteem needs are feeling good about what we bring to the world, whether it is through family, friends, work or our hobbies. Esteem needs mean that we each feel that we have value in our area of society. Finally, once esteem needs are met, we can seek to be self-actualized. A self-actualized person is typically one who is creative, inspired and often inspiring.

There is recognition that loss of any motivation level has wide effects, damaging all higher levels. For example, a person who loses their job will have a weakening of their esteem and their love until they can regain the safety provided by their work. Similarly, a person who loses a significant person in their life will not only have the love need impacted, but esteem and self-actualization, which depend on having love. This needs hierarchy is often represented as a pyramid, with the base made of the physical needs, and each level above resting on the level below.

# Vision

Like hearing and body senses (touch, temperature, etc.), vision uses a lobe of the brain, the occipital lobe in the back of the head, to make sense of what we see. Unlike the other senses, vision also has processing in the eye itself, to identify information before it gets to the brain, and our sense of vision uses many other brain regions to process the visual information after it has gone through the occipital lobe. For example, when we read words, the visual information of the words must be deciphered in the language comprehension area (Wernicke's area) in the temporal lobe and then this information goes to the speech area (Broca's area) in the frontal lobe. Also, we rely on a facial recognition area in the temporal lobe (a structure called the fusiform face area) to identify a face and its expression, with this region using mirror neurons to not only identify the expression but to mirror the feeling of it in our own minds.

## Optics of the Eye

The eye is a nearly spherical structure, with its shape made by the sclera and the cornea. The sclera is the tough white part eyeball, while the cornea is the clear part in front. The cornea, because of its shape, focuses light, with the lens inside the eye finishing this focus. Focusing of light by the cornea and lens is necessary to create an image on the retina, which is the light-sensitive part of the eye. The cornea and lens is similar to a camera lens, they create an image at the light-sensitive area. The cornea has a constant focusing strength and the lens is adjustable, letting us focus on things that are both near and far by changing the shape of the lens inside the eye.

Between the cornea and the lens is the iris. The iris provides an opening (the aperture of a camera) that controls the amount of light that enters the eye. The iris is pigmented (this pigment has many shades, giving us brown eyes, or hazel or blue, etc.), and the opening of the iris is called the pupil. This opening decreases in bright light and gets larger in dim light, to give us a wide range of light in which we can see.

## Cataracts

A cataract is when the lens of the eye becomes whiter instead of clear. Cataracts form in the lens due to exposure over many years to ionizing radiation, such as UV from the sun, microwaves or nuclear radiation. The energy in this high intensity radiation changes the structure of the proteins in the lens, modifying their structure, which makes them go from transparent to opaque. A similar thing happens when we cook an egg. Exposure to heat turns the transparent white of the egg into an opaque white structure. The best protection from cataracts is to keep UV away from your eyes with glasses that block all the UV, and wearing a hat or eyeshade that prevents the sunlight from directly reaching the eyes.

Once cataracts develop, the only solution currently is to remove the lens from the eye, since the cataract is in it, and to replace the lens with a plastic lens that will focus light. The disadvantage is the plastic lens can only focus at one distance, so glasses are needed to allow us to see at different distances. Cataracts typically develop later in life (after age fifty), since they are due to lifetime exposure to ionizing radiation.

## Glaucoma

Directly behind the cornea and in front of the iris is a fluid filled space called the aqueous humor. Fluid is constantly being filtered into this space, and it is constantly being drained from it, keeping this fluid perfectly clean. In certain medical conditions, the fluid does not drain well, and the excess fluid increases pressure in the eye. This occurs in many types of glaucoma, where there is a gradual increase in pressure in the eye. Glaucoma is treated with special eye drops that slow down the fluid production and protect from losing vision. An uncontrolled pressure increase causes a gradual loss of vision by damaging the optic nerve.

Glaucoma is an eye disease that usually affects people after age sixty. The best way to avoid it is to get eye pressure measured every year, so if the pressure begins to increase, it can be treated right away.

If glaucoma is not treated, a person gradually loses their vision, starting with loss of peripheral vision and moving toward the center. This means that the field of view gets more and more narrow with untreated glaucoma.

Other treatments for glaucoma may include certain medicinal plants that reduce eye pressure or protect the retinal cells from damage. The most common plant for this is marijuana, where the active ingredients are believed to reduce damage to the optic nerve (it is best to first discuss this with an ophthalmologist, who is an MD trained in eye diseases). If the fluid pressure does not decrease with medication, another solution is to put a tiny shunt in the eye to let a small amount of fluid leak out. This can only be done by a trained ophthalmologist who has experience with this type of surgery, and it can be very effective for these specific types of cases.

### Corrective Lenses

While the fluid of the aqueous humor helps maintain the structure and curvature of the cornea, it is the vitreous humor that maintains the full shape of the eyeball. The vitreous humor has a gelatin-like consistency and fills the majority of the eyeball behind the lens, keeping the round shape of the eye.

Optically, then, light passes through the cornea, aqueous humor, iris, lens and vitreous humor on its path to the retina, the light-sensitive part of the eye. The cornea and lens are the refractive (light-bending) parts, with the lens able to adjust the focus, and the iris regulates the amount of light that passes.

Any irregularity in the shape of the eye or of the cornea causes distortion of vision. When the cornea is not symmetrical, astigmatism results, meaning the focus at one angle differs slightly from the focus at another angle. If the overall shape of the cornea is rounder or flatter, then the conditions of myopia (near-sighted) or hyperopia (far-sighted) result, because the focus is being slightly different from what is needed to form a clear image on the retina. This means that slight changes in the shape of the cornea cause variations from normal focus.

### Presbyopia

As we age, the lens of the eye becomes less flexible and over many years gets less able to focus onto things that are close to us. This loss of flexibility means our nearest point of clear vision gets further away as we age. At twenty, the closest we can see something clearly is a distance of about 10 cm (2.5 inches). By forty the nearest we can see may be arms length, and then by sixty or seventy it can be a meter (three feet) away. This is why most need reading glasses after age forty, so they can focus on something they are holding.

For those who are myopic (near-sighted, or able to see near objects clearly but unable to focus clearly on distant objects), the decrease in lens flexibility has less effect than it does for others, simply because they started from a point closer to them. As they age, their vision seems to become more normal, and they can read without reading glasses for many years.

There are a few things to be aware of from this. First, near-sighted people can focus on something closer to their eyes than far-sighted people. Second, as we age, presbyopia moves the near point of vision further from our eyes. This is particularly noticeable over the age of fifty. For a normal sighted person (neither near nor far), the closest object one can see is about 10 cm at twenty years of age. By forty years, the nearest point of vision is about 20 cm, and at sixty years, the nearest point is about 80 cm, increasing to a full meter by seventy.

### Surgical Correction

For some who are strongly near-sighted, there is the possibility of reducing the need for glasses by reshaping the cornea in a surgical procedure. This process, called LASIK, changes the curvature of the cornea by cutting the cornea. The cuts to the cornea make it thinner, but they also allow the cornea to take a more optimal shape for normal vision. This does mean that the cornea becomes thinner, so the surgery cannot be repeated without risk of making the cornea too thin. If this were to happen, the cornea would not hold its shape, and the person would have vision that could not hold its focus well. This surgery does work well for 80 percent to 90 percent of those getting it (the problems are often with a difficulty in driving at night, as the cut cornea reflects lights, so oncoming traffic can be blinding), and they do not need glasses for distance. As presbyopia develops, however, they need glasses at an earlier age than if they had not had the surgery done.

### Retinal Function

Within the retina, there are two types of photoreceptors, the rod photoreceptors that provide for our night vision, and are exquisitely sensitive to very little light, and the cone photoreceptors that provide color vision. Each cone photoreceptor is sensitive to one of three colors, red, green or blue. The amounts of each of these three primary colors allow us to know the color of any object, and to see the full spectrum of the rainbow. This feature of only detecting three colors is why we can see all colors when we look at a computer display, which only has red, green and blue (RGB). It is also why we see all colors in a printed picture, which is typically made from cyan, magenta and yellow (the complementary colors to RGB). The central part of the retina, called the fovea, contains a very high number of cone photoreceptors packed into a very small space, which allows us to make out a lot of detail, which is called visual acuity.

The fovea provides this high acuity for the very middle (the central two degrees) of our visual field. Outside of the fovea, there is a mixture of rod and cone photoreceptors, and the acuity is reduced, though the sensitivity to low light levels is higher thanks to the rods. This is why on a moon-lit night, it is easier to see something when it is not straight in front of you, as the rod photoreceptors needed to see in dim light are not in the middle of our vision.

Inside the eyeball and behind the light-sensitive retina is a supportive tissue called the retinal pigmented epithelium (RPE). The RPE has two important roles, one optical and the other chemical. Optically, the RPE cells are black, and they surround the rods and cones. This means that any light that misses the photoreceptors is absorbed by the RPE and we have no reflections. This black curtain keeps us from seeing halos around objects, and so is essential for high acuity. In nocturnal animals, such as cats, the epithelium is reflective, allowing them to capture every bit of light. Because of this light reflection, their vision in dim light is very good, but their acuity is not as good as it is for us.

*Blind spot*

There is a spot in each eye where there are no rods or cones. This spot is where the optic nerve leaves the eye and where blood vessels enter and leave. The spot is called the blind spot, because we cannot see anything in that area. It is located on the nose side of the fovea by several millimeters, so the blind area is out to the sides for each eye. The area of the visual field that we are blind to is in different places for each eye. For the right eye it is about 15 degrees to the right, and for the left eye it is about 15 degrees to the left.

How is it that we do not notice this blind spot in our vision?

First, we have binocular, or 3-D, vision, meaning that each eye is conveying information about the same visual scene, but from a slightly different angle. This allows us to know the distance of things we see, but it also lets us fill in what is missing from one eye.

Second, even when we are looking with just one eye, our brain fills in when there is missing information. So, when we do not have information about a small space in our visual field, our brain fills this in with the same scene that we see next to the missing spot. For example, if the blind spot is looking toward the sky, the brain fills in the appropriate blue, and continues the cloud pattern that is right next to the spot. But, if we are looking at something that is only in the blind spot, it is invisible to us. You can test this with the diagram below. Close your left eye, and focus on the cross with your right eye. Move this page closer and further from your eye until the black dot on the right disappears. When it disappears, it is because it is in your blind spot.

Having this blind spot is a small disadvantage compared to the advantage of high acuity and fast vision that it allows us to have. The black-colored RPE uses vitamin A to recycle our rod and cone light-sensing chemicals. By having the RPE do this, the rods and cones work faster. And since the RPE puts a black screen behind these photoreceptors, we have clear vision.

## Macular Degeneration

Age-related macular degeneration (AMD) is a condition in which the retina is damaged in the central region, called the macula. The macula includes the fovea and the area around it, so damage reduces the high acuity central vision that we rely on for looking at things. AMD most commonly develops after age sixty, and lifestyle choices that reduce blood flow to the retina can increase the risk of developing AMD. This means that smoking, elevated cholesterol, high blood pressure, and lack of exercise increase risk of AMD. There is a genetic aspect as well, so if it is common in your family, it is important to have regular ophthalmological exams that look at the retina, eat a healthy diet with plenty of leafy green vegetables and fish, and keep physically active. Once AMD starts to develop, taking a supplement with vitamins C and E, zinc, beta-carotene or lutein and zeaxanthin slows the progress of this disease. These compounds are present in leafy greens and fish, and seem to only help as a supplement if the disease has already started. The specific amounts of each of these compounds is listed on the web site of the National Institutes of Health (nei.nih.gov), and many supplements follow the specific levels advised here, so it is important to know the amounts before choosing a supplement.

If AMD is advanced, there is another treatment to slow the progression of the disease. In most cases (90 percent) of AMD, vision is lost because blood capillaries grow on top of the retina. There are two ways to stop these vessels from growing without damaging the retina. The most common is a drug that selectively stops blood vessel growth. There are three drugs that are currently available to do this, Avastin, Lucentis and Eylea. Any one of these is injected into the eye, and it stops blood vessel growth for weeks or months at a time. Many people receiving these injections find that their vision does not get worse, and some find a small improvement.

# Cancer

We know a lot about cancer. For example, we know that it takes many mutations for a cell to become cancerous; we know that the body fights off most cancers before they get out of hand; we know about what can increase or decrease the risk of developing cancer; we know about genes that raise the risk of a cancer; and we know of treatments to reduce a cancer. But one thing we rarely discuss is why do some people avoid cancer while others get it? This is not an easy question, of course, because no one can be sure that they will never have cancer. But we can look at what we do know to help make sense of this, and to give all of us ways to reduce the risk of developing cancer.

To be absolutely clear: nobody can guarantee that someone will avoid cancer, and no one can guarantee that someone will get cancer. But we can be sure that certain things will reduce the risk of developing a cancer. And we can reduce this risk not by a few percent but we can cut the risk nearly in half, and cut it in half TWICE. Yes, we know things that will reduce a person's risk of cancer to about one quarter of the average. So by following certain practices, you can have a much better than average chance of a cancer free life.

## Epidemiology

We know a lot about cancer. And what we know about it, we've learned in a few ways. One way is with epidemiology. Epidemiology studies the spread of disease. This is when we look at what people eat, compare different foods in a diet, look at the different rates of each cancer, and learn which foods protect people from that cancer. There are people who spend their lives studying these relationships. We call them epidemiologists, and they have a lot of useful information for us about things that can help cause cancers and other things that can reduce cancers.

A way we learn about cancer is from statistics that epidemiologists have collected over the years. These statistics look at the number of people who have contracted specific cancers, and the number of people who have died from specific cancers. These numbers show trends among cancers in the country. A great example of this is the American Cancer Society's website <http://www.cancer.org>. On this site, under the Research header are "Cancer facts and figures." This page has links for many charts about cancer in the United States, including the incidence, by gender, for each cancer type and the deaths, by gender, for each cancer type. As you read these charts, some things are clear. For example, it is easy to see the link between smoking and cancer and recognize that there is a delay of twenty to twenty-five years from a change in smoking to a similar change in cancer. This convinces us that smoking causes cancer, and that it takes (on average) twenty to thirty years to make those cancers. So, smoking for a couple of decades is life threatening, but smoking for a short time (months or a year or two) is something you can more likely recover from. The challenge here, of course, is that smoking is addictive, and as with any addition, we develop a dependence on the drug, making it extremely difficult to quit. But if you smoke, know that quitting will improve your health.

### Experimentation

Another method that has been used to learn about cancer has been laboratory experiments. Experiments use cancer cells grown in controlled conditions. These cancer cells come from a human cancer and they continue to grow in a lab setting as long as nutrients are provided. One stunning fact about cancer cells is that they can continue to grow and multiply indefinitely. In 1951 a small bit of cancer was removed from a woman and grown in a solution providing basic nutrients. This small piece of cancer has grown to be twenty tons today, and it continues to be used in research on cancer. We have learned a great deal from just this one cancer, so much so that there are now 11,000 U.S. patents that used these cells. (The story has been well described in the book, *The Immortal Life of Henrietta Lacks*, by R. Skloot).

Cancer cells grown in a laboratory can be tested to learn what may slow or stop the cancer. This is how drugs are first tested to learn what affects the cancer and also how we can stop it.

What we have learned about cancer is that normal cells in our body become pre-cancerous from time to time. This is common, and it occurs in everyone. Usually our immune system destroys these pre-cancerous cells, and healthy cells replace them. Occasionally, one of these pre-cancerous cells become cancerous. Again the immune system usually eliminates it before it becomes a problem. But on rare occasions one of these cancerous cells is able to multiply and become a small tumor. If we detect it early, we can have it removed. But if it is hidden, it may grow to be large, it may metastasize. In either case it begins to affect us in more harmful ways.

### What is cancer

A cancer is a group of cells that have acquired new characteristics and create a tumor. The term was coined by Hippocrates (460-370 BC) to describe the crab-like structure of these tumors, with arms coming out of the tumor and going into the body tissue around it. The key new characteristic is the ability to reproduce without a limit. This feature of cancer means that the cancer cells can divide repeatedly, growing a tumor, so long as they have a blood supply. In normal body cells, there is a limit to the number of times a cell can divide. The limit is because of the structure of our DNA. Every time a cell divides, a little of the DNA at the end of the chromosome is cut off, almost like a handle for the chromosome that detaches. This DNA at the ends of the chromosomes is called a telomere. The telomere is a small bit of DNA at the end of a chromosome, and a little of it is lost with each cell division. The rest of the DNA carries the genes that code for the cell components, so no information is lost. But with each cell division, the telomeres get shorter, and eventually the telomere is gone (after fifty to eighty cell divisions). After that, the cell cannot divide any more. The only exception to this are cells that replace the telomere. Cancer cells are able to replace the telomere, and can keep making new cells.

Cancer cells have other mutations, including ones that keep the immune system from killing them, and making blood vessels grow into the tumors to feed them.

### How cells become cancerous

This makes for quite a few new abilities needed for a cell to become a cancer. It has been estimated that a cell needs five or six mutations to become cancerous. These mutations are each changes to the DNA. Any one change is not harmful to a person, but all together they are dangerous.

With all the mutations that need to occur, developing a cancer takes time. In fact, it can take decades for cancer to develop. There are several reasons why cancer is rare. First is DNA itself. As a cell divides, the copying of DNA also checks to make sure there are no errors. When some mutations happen, the cell repairs the DNA right away. So cell division is not usually a source of mutations.

The next protection is after a mutation has happened. If one cell is has a mutation and is now working differently, the cells around it instruct it to sacrifice itself for the good of the whole body, or the immune system kills it directly. This protection keeps the vast majority of mutated cells from surviving, and protects us from most pre-cancers developing. Unfortunately, if the mutation of the pre-cancerous cell ignores these cell signals, the cell can grow and divide, giving the mutation a chance to keep on.

Once a cell has acquired most of the mutations needed to be cancerous, this cancerous cell can make copies of itself, gradually creating a small lump of identical cancer cells, called a tumor, or a cancer *in situ* (a cancer that is staying in place). At this stage, it is only dangerous if it develops the other mutations to become malignant (bad). Otherwise it could stay as an *in situ* cancer forever. If it does acquire further mutations, it can then reach the state of a cancer: dividing without control, not responding to external signals, getting its own blood supply, and even leaving its location and making tumors elsewhere in the body.

Once these properties are acquired, there is a tumor and it is capable of spreading (metastasizing) to other regions of the body. The tumor can grow rapidly, and will make new blood vessels grow and support it.

A comparison of these cancer and normal cell traits is listed in the table below.

| Normal Cells | Cancer Cells |
|---|---|
| Limited number of cell divisions | Unlimited cell division |
| Controlled growth | Uncontrolled growth |
| Socially well behaved (normal interactions with other cells) | Selfish. Do not respond to signals from other cells, and have blood vessels grow to them |
| No telomerase | Produce telomerase (an enzyme that maintains the telomere) |
| Need blood nutrients to grow | Grow with fewer nutrients |
| Exhibit contact inhibition (growth is curtailed when pushed on by adjacent cells) | No contact inhibition |
| Normal karyotype (normal number and shape of chromosomes) | Polyploid and/or aneuploidy (many or few chromosomes, and unusual shapes) |
| | Cause cancer when injected into mice |

### How Cancers are Terminated

As long as a cancer has a blood supply, it can keep growing. This need for blood led to a cancer therapy using a drug that blocks new blood vessel growth. The cancer drug Avastin is one that works in this way, and was the first cancer drug that stopped the blood supply rather than killing cells that were dividing. This starves a tumor, killing the rapidly dividing cells, and shrinking a tumor. This is not a wonder drug, however, as each cancer can be resistant to one set of drugs and succumb to another. Other ways of reducing tumor size include surgery, where the larger masses can be removed, and radiation, which acts by mutating the cancer so that it dies.

### What We've Learned

We have learned that cancers usually come about slowly, taking many years for a normal cell to become cancerous. We learned that this requires at least five mutations in a cell before it becomes cancerous. Also, research has shown that mutations are more likely when cells are stressed. This stress can be from an irritant (such as smoking, which irritates the lungs, making the irritated cells mutate). If those mutations continue, which is very likely if there is continued irritation, then the mutant cells may grow more quickly. With more time, these can become cancerous.

Fortunately, our body's immune system usually catches an early mutation and destroys it, so while we are always developing very early pre-cancers, the vast majority of them are eliminated. This process is helped by what strengthens the immune system: a healthy diet, regular exercise and sleep, and not smoking.

### Decreasing Our Cancer Risk

Overall, we want to reduce exposure to irritants to decrease mutations, and eliminate mutations as quickly as possible.

This latter point is key. If a cell mutates and is pre-cancerous or cancerous, it may take months or years for it to become a large enough tumor to cause pain. In fact, most cancer does not cause pain, but is noticed because it does something, perhaps pushing or blocking a normal action in another part of the body. But it takes time for this to happen. Even if cells are dividing rapidly, it will take dozens of cell divisions before there is a tumor the size of a pencil point, but then just a dozen more divisions will make it the size of an olive, and another dozen could make it as big as a fist. So catching it early is critical. Since it is hard to detect a cancer at these earliest stages, we have to rely on our body to catch and destroy them. Once a cancer is large enough to detect, it is usually causing other problems.

Let's look at what we can do.

Anything we do that helps our body prevent a cancer from occurring, or eliminate a new cancer, improves our chances of a healthy life. Most things we do help our body prevent or fight cancer involves diet and exercise. And these two make a huge difference, being able to reduce our risk to one quarter. The only other things that will reduce our risk dramatically are reducing our exposure to carcinogens and being born with the right genes. While we can control exposure to a degree, we cannot control genes. But we can control diet and exercise. And in doing so we not only take charge of our own health, we have the biggest impact on living a healthy life.

Finally, whether we like it or not, this is an odds game at some point: If you happen to get cancer it simply means you did not win on those odds, as so many find out. You can reduce your odds, but you cannot guarantee not getting cancer. If you do get cancer and you've been following all this advice, you will likely have a better chance of joining the ranks of cancer survivors.

# Health Sustaining Actions

There are many things that we do each day that affect our long-term health. In fact, the biggest effect on our health is from our patterns of daily living. These patterns include our choices of food, activity, and lifestyle. These everyday choices, and not the occasional big celebration feast, have the biggest effect on our health.

Another thing that impacts our health is getting regular medical checkups, including screening for cancer and heart disease. The reason is that the survival odds for any medical condition is much higher when a disease is found early. Other aspects of life, such as exposure to toxins in our environment (home, work, or play) or the genes we have inherited also play a role, and offer a caution of what we may need to do to reduce damage to our bodies. These latter ones are things we often learn about after the fact, so while it is wise not to grow up in an area with toxins that may affect you, we usually learn about such a thing after we've lived there, so this reminds us to be watchful. As for the genes, if many of our direct relatives have a particular medical condition, then it is more likely that we may get it as well, and this lets us know to modify our food and activity to help reduce our risk.

In terms of the first three items, chapters on foods and physical activity follow this chapter. The points about lifestyle are discussed in this chapter. The biggest health effect from lifestyle choices is smoking. We know from countless studies that the foods we eat, the level of physical activity we engage in, and whether we are non-smokers has a huge effect on our physical health, our risk of many diseases, and our productive lifespan.

## No Smoking

Smoking is hazardous to our health because it increases the risk for cancer, heart disease, and lung disease. The smoke itself is dangerous because of the tiny particles in it (and yes, any smoke is dangerous), but smoking is also dangerous because of the chemicals in the tobacco (which makes cigarette smoking as well as vaping especially hazardous). All smoke is harmful to us, reducing lung capacity and causing inflammation in the lungs that can lead to cancer or other lung diseases.

The reason it is strongly recommended never to smoke is because of these health risks, but also because smoking is addictive. Once someone takes up the habit of smoking, the addictive nature of cigarettes makes it very hard to quit. For this reason, it is best never to smoke. If you do smoke, it is important to begin today to take steps to reduce it, with a goal of quitting. The key is to treat each day as a goal – to reduce your smoking today. And then to do it again tomorrow, for each day is a new opportunity, and each day you have a good chance to succeed. Keep that in mind, and make the effort today.

## Alcohol

Alcohol has positive and negative effects on us, with the positives only in limited amounts. There are several things we know about alcohol. It has a lot of calories (calories is a measure of food energy) but they are "empty calories" (meaning there is no nutritional value). We also know that alcohol is toxic for the brain of a developing fetus or young child, so pregnant women should try not to drink any alcohol and small children should not be given alcohol.

We also know that some wines may be cardio-protective when used in moderation (moderation being about one glass of wine a day for an average-sized person. This effect seems to be true for red wines, though there is also information that this may not be helpful for women who are of childbearing years.

Wine has the same calories as any other alcohol, but the nutrients in the grapes may give us some heart benefit. However, the additional calories cause our body to grow (this is why we have the term "beer belly"). When our body has too much growth energy, we risk two things: gaining weight that puts stress on our heart and may lead to type II diabetes and an increased cancer risk. So, while a glass of red wine may have a modest benefit, more is harmful for our health.

Another concern about alcohol is that alcohol is toxic for our body. Our liver detoxifies chemicals such as alcohol that get into our body. The toxins are eliminated, but the liver itself can be damaged by exposure to the toxins. Also, the speed of the liver in detoxifying alcohol varies from person to person. Some individuals have very active alcohol dehydrogenase and others have less. If you feel the effect of alcohol quickly, you have low levels, which means that alcohol stays in your body longer and has a stronger effect on your thinking process and a harder effect on your organs. A simple rule to know how alcohol is affecting you is have someone observe your ability to move accurately. If you are clumsy, you have had more alcohol than advisable. If this lasts for a while (more than an hour), then your organs are more affected by this much alcohol.

Overall, it seems that when choosing to drink, all alcohol should be consumed in moderation, with one or perhaps two drinks per day, and no binge drinking. Consumption of a large amount of alcohol at once is dangerous. It puts a lot of stress on your body, and it is a signal for some cancers.

## *Drugs*

Drugs also have many effects on us. Whether the drugs are medicinal or psychotropic, they all change our normal body function, posing risks for us. Again, moderation may make the most sense. If it is a drug to treat a medical condition, then use it as prescribed, and no more. Failure to use it can harm you, overuse can cause other effects, so following the recommendation for medical use is best. If it is a drug that affects your brain, and you wish to use it for the mood effect, it is wise to do so under supervision, and to be very cautious to use the smallest amount that works. This is especially true for opioid drugs, for two critical reasons. First, opioids are strongly addictive, and it is very difficult to quit them once addition begins. Opioid addition can begin within a couple of weeks of taking these drugs, so if you are prescribed them for pain, it should not be for more than a week or ten days. Of course, pain treatment is extremely difficult, and this should only be done under a doctor's supervision. As far as you can, work to avoid opioid drugs and limit use to a week. The second caution about opioids is that they have more than one effect. The first effect is the analgesia (pain relief) that allows someone to feel good. But the second effect is to reduce respiration (breathing). With higher levels of opioids, we not only feel fine, but our breathing slows and can stop. The extreme danger is that someone addicted to opioid drugs may have taken a dose of the drug that not only makes them high, but slows their breathing. If this happens, it is urgent to get medical care immediately. There is a treatment drug called naloxone (brand name Narcan) that can be used to stop the opioid action, and let breathing restart. This needs to be given to someone before they suffocate.

So with drugs, as with alcohol, moderation is key, using as little as possible, and being particularly cautious with drugs that are addictive. With prescription medication for infections or virulent disease, adhere closely to the recommendations.

## Sugar

We have a vast amount of refined sugar available to us every day. We know that sugar is a carbohydrate, and it is present in most foods to some extent. In most natural foods, we have complex carbohydrates, rather than simple sugar, and our digestive system takes more time to break apart the complex carbohydrate so our cells can use it. This digestion time gives us a big advantage as complex carbohydrates give us a slow release of sugar into our body to provide energy for hours, rather than the immediate energy burst from refined sugar, which quickly fades.

Many fruits have sugar in its more simple form, but the sugar is mixed with other compounds to create the flavor of the fruit and to give our body nutrients that help us. With all the refined sugar in foods today, we find ourselves eating sugar much more than our ancestors did. Sugar today is added to many foods and drinks, and to such an extent that estimates are we are consuming more than ten times the sugar that society did long ago. U.S. per-capita sugar consumption has gone from under 5 kg per year 200 years ago to 50 kg per year now, and China is now seeing a large increase each year in sugar consumption.

Many studies have indicated that this excess sugar harms our bodies. First, all the sugar needs to be digested and stored. The next problem is that by eating refined sugar, we consume more calories each day than we need, so we store it as fat (adipose tissue). The swings in blood sugar put more stress on our kidneys to filter this out, while the increase in body weight and extra fat makes our heart work harder, raising our blood pressure. Increases in sugar and in body weight also increase our risk for developing Type II diabetes. The increase in sugar and fat will also increase our risk of cancer, because the sugar provides more energy for early cancer cells to grow, and the fat sends out signals telling cells, including cancer cells, to take in more sugar and increase in number. For these reasons, reducing consumption of refined sugar, whether in prepared foods, drinks, desserts, or elsewhere, is an important step in improving our long-term health.

## Medical Exams and Genetics

Keeping up with regular medical exams is important for good health. With each visit to a health care practitioner, it is useful to be ready to ask questions. For example, if you have a change in a mole on your skin, or a sudden change in weight, or you find yourself out of breath often, ask your health practitioner what these may be due to, what you should look for, and what may need urgent attention. Having an understanding of how your body works helps, as you are the one person who knows your body well. For this reason, it is important for you to be aware of your body, of any changes, and of what symptoms may indicate you need a checkup.

Included in the regular medical exams is the need for regular dental exams. We now know that bacteria in our teeth and gums increases our risk of heart disease. This means daily brushing and flossing of our teeth and regular dental exams reduce our risk of heart disease.

Knowing your family health history also helps you know possible conditions you may be at risk for. While we can test for the genes that confer some risks, the easiest way to understand all conditions you may be at risk for is to talk with your extended family and learn all the medical conditions any direct relative has. If a lot of your relatives have a particular condition, it is likely that you are at risk for it. And since most conditions are due to both genetics and what we do, when you are aware that you are at risk, you will be able to take action to lower your odds of contracting the condition. For example, if a third of your relatives have type II diabetes, then it would be ideal for you to have regular exercise and a healthy diet to keep your body weight in the normal range, and avoid snacks made of high fat or high carb foods. We know that those at risk for type II diabetes are less likely to suffer from it if they have a normal body weight, a lot of exercise and a moderate diet. Being aware of your family history can reduce your odds of developing diabetes.

# Activity

Being active improves your odds of avoiding cancer or heart disease. When we are active, we use some of the nutrients in our blood to make energy for our muscles, so they don't create plaque in the arteries or get stored in fat tissue. In using these instead, we decrease the growth signals given by fat cells, which means cancer cells are not stimulated, and we also make sure our heart does not get overworked. Improving blood flow improves efficiency as well, and our muscles more easily get the nutrients they need.

This means that by being active, you have lower odds of getting heart disease or cancer. In fact, the cancer risk is almost cut in half by being active. Few things in life have such a great payback. Here is how you can increase your odds of winning in your fight against cancer and heart disease: Be active.

The biggest questions about this always seem to relate to how much activity, what kinds of activity, and how strenuous this activity needs to be. First the good news: The activity can be any kind of movement, including walking, and it should be a minimum of thirty to forty minutes a day, and ideally sixty minutes per day. This means that if you walk twice a day for twenty minutes each time, your activity is helpful. A little more helps, but the biggest improvement is that first thirty to forty minutes of moderate exercise each day. The exercise does not need to be strenuous. A good walk is enough. Normal daily activities like doing the wash, cleaning, gardening, also add to a more active lifestyle.

Making the exercise a part of your normal activities makes a big difference. It is important simply to get up and move. Ideally, the movement should be at the level of a brisk walk (or more), but the movement is the key part. If you make it part of your daily routine, it is much better than if you try to remember to do it once in a while, because the regularity is important.

If you wonder how much more is helpful, know that while the first half hour gives the greatest benefit, a little more time or a little more vigorous exercise is also beneficial. Getting in thirty minutes of vigorous exercise (running, swimming, etc.) is great for you, as all the exercises that improve your cardiovascular system also improve your odds of being disease free. The important thing is to keep at it. If you normally have a vigorous workout and cannot do so for a period of time, consider taking walks to keep up your regular activity level. This will help you keep to your routine, and continue your health benefit from activity.

For those trying to find thirty minutes to walk each day, there are several creative solutions. Some people eat lunch while walking around or even walking inside a building or parking lot. Others use their coffee breaks as time to get in a short walk (ten minutes), and then make time to walk an extra ten minutes after work. Still others may park farther from work, or exit the transit system a stop early to make sure they get in a walk, while others come to work early in order to take a swimming break when the local pool opens in the afternoon. Each of us needs to find the type of activity we enjoy. Sometimes it is easier to do it with a friend, or as a continuation of a sport you enjoy (an afternoon game or swim or run). An excellent resource for ideas is to talk about it with people you know, as you may find an activity partner or someone who will encourage you in your efforts.

Since any exercise done regularly will reduce your disease risk, it is valuable to get started. Try something! If it does not motivate you to do it regularly, try something else. Try different things to get the exercise in, as variety can help keep us going, and can help us find what we like best.

Be aware that the type of activity will change with your interests and age. Each of us has certain things we enjoy and if we have those things as our regular activity, that helps us.

Why is it that activity helps us so much with cancer and heart disease? Certainly reducing the chance of developing cancer by half is a huge difference. From what we have been learning about cancer, we are finding that pre-cancers, or cancer-like cells, develop fairly commonly in us, but our own immune system stops these, and exercise helps the immune system. Physical activity reduces our stress and improves our cardiovascular system as well as our mental condition. All of these make a difference in how well our immune system performs. When we are stressed, our immune system is suppressed. In contrast, when we are content or happy, our immune system does well. And when we keep our heart and blood vessels working smoothly, then all the body's systems are more efficient, and this helps our immune system work better.

So, all kinds of activity help our immune system, and that substantially reduces our chance of developing cancer or heart disease.

# Food

Just as regular exercise makes a big difference in our health, so does good food. A healthy diet reduces our chance of getting cancer by half, and substantially lowers our risk of heart disease. This is a bit more confusing than the activity rule for better health, as what makes up a healthy diet changes as we learn more about the effect of different foods.

So, where do we start? To eat healthy means many things. Let's start with the overall concept. Our diet is what we eat, and includes all the foods we eat. This includes a variety of things, all of which are important in the overall diet. These things include what foods are eaten, how much of each we eat, and how often we eat. Some aspects involve our eating schedule: whether we eat a lot at once, starve regularly, have three meals a day, and so on. Other aspects include balance in the diet itself: Do you eat fruits and vegetables each day or infrequently, what kinds of protein or carbohydrates or fats are in your diet, do you eat a lot of artificial compounds, or processed foods, or locally grown foods?

The challenge is that the concept of a healthy diet is always changing as we learn more. One rule of thumb is everything in moderation. When you learn that dark chocolate has antioxidants that are good for you, it means that dark chocolate *in moderation* is good in a healthy diet. Moderation may mean 25 grams (1 oz.) in a day, but it also includes being aware that this same chocolate may have additional fats and sugars that affect how much you should eat. So, while an ounce or two of chocolate may be fine, a pound (half kilo) in one day is not. In the same manner, while one glass of red wine may be beneficial in a daily diet, a bottle of wine is not. So, moderation is important. Each food that has compounds that are good for us may also include some that are bad in greater amounts (like the sugars and fats with chocolate or the alcohol in wine). But this also makes the work of choosing foods more of a challenge (as well as potentially more fun).

How do we get some guidance on this? There are many web sites that give nutritional advice, and ones that are from established medical research institutions are most careful to be accurate. They are very good resources to learn what the current understanding of nutrition is. For example, the National Institutes of Health maintains an extensive site of information (www.nih.gov), as does the Mayo Clinic (www.mayoclinic.com), the American Cancer Society (www.cancer.org) and the American Heart Association (www.heart.org). There are many other reputable sites, but these four alone have a lot of current information that can be helpful. A good way to gauge information is to compare it with what is in the NIH site, as NIH is the governmental agency that manages medical research in the United States, and presents this information for the public.

To understand what we should be eating, let's think about the purposes of food. And there are many purposes! Food, of course, provides us with the materials and energy we need for each day. The materials include proteins and minerals and vitamins. And the energy is usually in the form of carbohydrates (like rice or corn or pasta or bread) or fats (from meats or oils, typically). Another purpose of food is emotional, sharing food when we are with others, or eating certain foods to feel better.

With regard to food, we are in a different place than our great grandparents were. A century or more ago, most people had to labor physically each day in their work and transit, so their bodies used more energy in a day than we use. At the same time, we have easy access to all kinds of foods. In each case (us and our ancestors), our bodies are designed for storing excess energy to use later, but today we rarely need this stored energy, since we can nearly always find food when we are hungry. This means that the stored energy in our bodies is converted to body fat, which is a great way to store energy for days or weeks, but is harmful when it is never used. Since we are less active than our ancestors, we do not need to use this fat in a normal week, so it stays and causes heart disease and type II diabetes, and increases our cancer risk.

To keep our energy in balance, eating the amount we use, most of us need to eat less and exercise more. Doing one without the other does not work for long, but the two together work very well, and help bring our body into balance.

Why do many of us have a hard time keeping a constant weight? There are many reasons. We often have stress in our lives or work, which makes us seek out foods that are comforting. Another reason is that our metabolism slows as we get older, so a person of forty or fifty needs less food than the same person did at age twenty. Other reasons can be less time for exercise, or eating snacks mindlessly.

With our body optimized to store energy and our taste enjoying the flavor of fat and sugar, we have to be careful and watch what we are eating to keep from getting out of balance. To make this harder, we are surrounded with so many tasty treats all the time and stress leads us to eat to keep alert or to be polite or to be calm.

As we have said, one way to compensate for this, and reduce stress, is to exercise. This helps in many ways: It gives us the physical activity our body needs for health, it lowers our stress, it uses some of the energy we have eaten, and it is harder to eat fatty foods after exercising. In the previous chapter we learned that physical activity improves our odds of being cancer-free, and now we see that it can help us eat a healthy diet.

So part of our role in diet is to be aware of what we are eating. Try to reduce or eliminate late snacks and do not eat between meals, as these habits increase the chance of getting type II diabetes, since it lets our body adapt to insulin, as explained in the diabetes chapter.

### How to revise your diet

Making changes to what we eat and keeping to this revised diet is about preparing healthy foods that you enjoy. The key aspect is finding foods you like, because we keep eating the foods we enjoy. A good way to enjoy the foods we should be eating is to make the meals we like from our childhood, but make small changes in them to reduce fats and meats, and increase vegetables. Another idea is to try out recipes, especially ones that use ingredients that are in abundance (when local farms have lots of something, then it is likely to be fresh and tasty). Modifying familiar recipes and taking on new ones where you like the foods are good ways to adjust your overall diet to provide healthier meals for you and your family.

Through this, develop meals that you like and that become the familiar foods for you. If you have children, involving them in the process usually helps keep them interested in the foods and gives you the chance to teach them at the same time. Seeing your desire to have your family eat healthily can then be part of how they learn the importance of a good diet.

### How to decide on your diet

Despite having more than enough protein and fat and

carbohydrates in our food, many of us do not get enough vitamins and minerals. Choosing foods that include many vegetables and fruits, especially if these are local and not processed, is a good way to get the vitamins and minerals and other plant compounds that keep us healthy. For example, we know that antioxidants are generally good for us, and we can get them in foods or in pills. But the pill includes just some antioxidants (perhaps vitamins C and E), and does not have the diversity of antioxidants that are found in nature. Simply eating a variety of fruits in a day gives more than just the few vitamins, it means we get a broad collection of vitamins and minerals, and studies have found that eating these in foods is more useful than from pills.

## How to decide on your diet – fats

There are many things to consider in choosing your overall diet. While there are a lot of claims for one diet or other, the best diet is the one we will keep to. And the diet we keep is the one we like the taste of and like how we feel on it. Many people enjoy a Mediterranean diet, or a fish diet, or vegan diet, and each of these can be fine for you. One thing common in each of these is a lower amount of red meat and animal fat and a higher amount of nutrients from vegetables and plant and/or fish oils. We do know that this is generally good for us: to eat less animal fats and increase plant and fish fats (oils). Animal fats are dangerous for our blood vessels and for our overall health, while fish and plant fats are better for our health. Even here, there are exceptions, hydrogenated plant oils are not good for us, so use plant oils that are monounsaturated or polyunsaturated (the saturated fats that come from animals and some plants are more of a problem for our bodies). Saturated fats increase our body low density lipoproteins (LDL) while the monounsaturated and polyunsaturated oils increase our highdensity lipoproteins (HDL). It is this LDL/HDL balance in our body that relates to heart health, with a lower LDL and higher HDL being best. Also, saturated fats give us a greater risk of cancer, as the the inflammation from them helps cancer to start.

## How to decide on your diet – calories

The total amount of calories (energy) we eat is important. Keeping our weight in a normal range and relatively constant lowers the risk of diabetes and cancer. Since we use less energy as we get older, we usually need to decrease how much we eat over the years. One useful trick is to pause while eating. Remember that it takes a while (about twenty minutes) for your brain to know that you've eaten. This is why we don't feel full until after we eat. Taking our time with a meal, or simply stopping, are ways to keep in balance.

## How to decide on your diet – chemicals

We regularly hear about the dangers of pesticides and some fertilizers in our foods. The reason they are dangerous is that many of these chemicals are mutagens or metabolic stimulants. The mutagens increase the risk of cancer. The stimulants increase the growth of our cells, which can increase our risk for many diseases. It is best to wash fruits and vegetables and to try to eat food that has no chemicals used in production.

If you use local, organically grown foods in season, you lower exposure to these chemicals and also get foods that have not lost nutrients from shipping. Local and organic foods have more nutrients and fewer toxins.

Other chemicals get into some foods in the preparation process. Some chemicals are for taste (smoke flavor or flavor enhancers), some for keeping foods fresher (preservatives), and some for food appearance (colors and the chemicals that create textures). If you can, try to minimize these. While each is tested for safety before it is used, there are so many in our diet that there is no way to know if the mix of all of them hurts us. Also, our bodies do not have a way to process most of these chemicals, so our liver needs to detoxify them to prevent damage to our cells. By reducing these chemicals there is less stress on your liver and kidneys.

### How to decide on your diet – fresh fruits and vegetables

Fresh fruits and vegetables have many nutrients that are good for us. These include the minerals and vitamins and fiber in these foods. These also include the many antioxidants and phytonutrients (nutrients from plants), some of which are described in the next chapter. Getting a variety of these in your daily diet is generally a good thing. And when we eat them, it is always best to eat them in a less processed manner. So, for example, carrot sticks are better for us than carrot cake, and an orange is better than orange juice from a carton.

Above all, try to find a diet that you enjoy. It may take time to develop and become used to it, but if you like this diet, you will be able to keep with it, and that makes all the difference.

# Beneficial Foods

The understanding of foods that are good for us is constantly changing because new studies continue to give us a more clear view. But food is the topic that can make a big difference for us in having a healthy and productive life. While there seems to always be someone claiming that a particular food does wonders in preventing heart disease or diabetes or cancer, the reality is that there is no magical food. While some foods are beneficial and others are not, no one has found a food that by itself has the power to cure. All studies show that a balance of a variety of beneficial foods is best, as long as we decrease the more harmful ones. The good news is that we can have a varied diet, and in fact, that is our best choice.

Overall, eating more fruits and vegetables, along with certain oils, is helpful. It reduces our risk for cancer, heart disease and diabetes, and it also helps in other ways by providing a better overall sense of fitness (feeling better about yourself and so being more active and interactive) as well as a better mood and visual appearance. The risk reduction may be due to the antioxidants and fiber in these fruits and vegetables, and to the decreased inflammation they provide.

So, what is best to eat more of, and which foods should we reduce or even avoid? There are some clear patterns: Eat less red meats and burnt foods (like barbecue), and eat more vegetables, fruits and fish. The reason is that foods that have more antioxidants or plant-based nutrients or fiber or omega-3 oils give us distinct benefits by preventing damage in our body. In contrast, foods that increase inflammation in our bodies are harmful. These harmful foods include ones that are higher in carcinogens such as charred fats (in barbecued meats), or that are more difficult for our bodies to process so our digestive tract is affected by the irritants for a long time (meats). This means that a more plant-based diet gives us an advantage.

### Eating Patterns and Habits – How to Succeed

A diet with variety is good, as we get a mix of beneficial foods, and it is this variety that makes the difference, as the combination works better than specific foods. It is the mixture of the vitamins and other plant nutrients that benefit our bodies, and not just one or two things. This may be why taking nutrients in pill form is not as useful as getting these same vitamins from foods, because the whole foods have other compounds that work together with the "active"ingredients to benefit our bodies.

Know that the best way for you to choose foods is to work with what you like, and then modify some parts of it to make it healthier. For example, in a Mediterranean diet, which is often found to be healthy, meats are used as a flavoring for a meal that includes a lot of vegetables rather than as the main food source. An example would be a meal for a family that uses 100-200 grams (about 1/3 pound) of meat that is cooked with onions or garlic and to which a kilogram or more (2-3 pounds) of chopped vegetables are added, all of which may be served with rice. Making modifications in foods you already like, where you reduce the meat and increase the vegetables while keeping the same spicing, will mean you and your family will continue to like the food and so will keep to this modified diet. This is true for adults and children. While our children often like the same foods, by making small changes to reduce meats and increase vegetables, they and we will both have a better diet to grow on.

Making dietary changes is hard. Most of us who make big changes in our diet switch back. But making smaller changes has been successful for many. It keeps the flavors that we prefer from our traditions, and simply modifies the preparation to increase our health benefit. As we adjust to the change, this new version becomes preferred. For example, reducing meat and increasing vegetables will mean less saturated fat. Once we've adjusted to this lower animal fat, having a meal with the higher fat feels less comfortable as we notice how much slower we move after eating it.

Overall, then, try to eat plants and use plant fats (oil) rather than animal fats, choosing from a variety of vegetables that are local and in season, and eating meals that you like (the animal exception is fish - eating a serving or two of fish each week is beneficial). Doing this will benefit you doubly: once by the healthier diet and second because it will be easy to keep to it.

These next sections are to give you more detail about what we know about various foods. But keeping to the guideline above is the key to a healthy diet.

### Foods to Increase – Berries

Berries are beneficial. We know that anthocyanins, which give blueberries and raspberries their color, are powerful antioxidants. These anthocyanins kill many types of cancer cells without harming us.

While most fruits have anthocyanins, foods with a lot of these compounds are berries. A simple rule to know if anthocyanins are in a fruit is to check the color: If a fruit has a strong red or purple color, it has these powerful compounds. Examples include berries, red grapes, red apples, peaches, cherries, and so on.

An easy way to increase your consumption of these foods is to have fresh fruit available in your home, choosing what is local and in season to maximize the nutrient content, or having frozen fruits available to thaw and eat. Locally grown fruits that are in season have been found to have higher amounts of the beneficial nutrients, and they also have more flavor (possibly because those "good" compounds provide flavor). The locally grown advantage seems to be because the fruit is picked ripe (which means more nutrients) and also because the freshest picked fruits have more nutrients (those compounds decrease a little each day).

You can use dried fruits (without added sugar) as a treat that provides the nutritional benefit, or purchase frozen berries that you can use in meals or mix into fruit drinks. Children often like a fruit drink or smoothie made by blending together a variety of fruits. To get the most benefit, do not add any sugars or ice cream, just use the fruit.

Anthocyanins are only one of the valuable compounds in fruits. Some others are carotenoids (which are yellow, orange and red in color and are strong antioxidants), polyphenols (these compounds may help our memory), and bioflavonoids, compounds that increase the antioxidant power of other molecules.

These compounds all seem to work best in combination, so consuming them by eating a variety of fruits may be advantageous over trying to take them in pill form.

### Foods to Increase – Cruciferous Vegetables

Another beneficial food category is cruciferous vegetables, also called *Brassica*. Cruciferous vegetables are in the cabbage family, and include broccoli, cauliflower, cabbage, kale and bok choy, among others. Studies have shown that these foods contain an anti-cancer compound called sulphoraphane. Sulphoraphane kills cancer cells in a different way from the anthocyanins mentioned above. Sulphoraphane dissolves in water, so we lose some of it when we boil these vegetables, with about half left after ten to fifteen minutes of boiling.

### Foods to Increase – Carotenoids

Carrots and tomatoes are full of carotenoids that give these foods their color and give us a health benefit. The carotenoids (beta-carotene in carrots, lycopene in tomatoes, and lutein in other fruits) are strong antioxidants that remove free-radicals in our cells, reducing inflammation and reducing the oxidation that can occur. This oxidation reduction can damage DNA, resulting in a mutation that could cause cancer. Beta-carotene is also used to make vitamin A. This vitamin is needed by our eyes to see light. Vitamin A is made from beta-carotene, and not from other carotenoids. Vitamin A is very important in our diet, and it is better to get it from food than a pill, as it is a vitamin that can cause damage if we take too much (skin damage and possibly liver damage). Consuming foods that are rich in carotenoids gives us ample vitamin A without risk of an overload. Also, by eating foods that have carotenoids, we get related compounds that are in these foods that provide other advantages for our body. When we primarily get our vitamins in pill form, we miss out on the other nutrients in food that our bodies need to maximize our health.

There are quite a few other foods with carotenoids, and these are foods that are orange and yellow-orange in color. The foods with the highest concentration of beta-carotene are carrots, pumpkin and sweet potato. These contain about ten times as much beta-carotene as the next foods on this list, which are also high in this nutrient. This next part of the list includes mango, kale, apricot, red bell pepper, cantaloupe, spinach, guava, broccoli, watermelon and Brussels sprouts.

### Foods to Increase – Fiber

Pectin is a complex carbohydrate, a soluble fiber, which is present in all fruits and vegetables, especially in their peels. It is highest in apple and peach peel, and is in high amounts in legumes (beans), whole grains, citrus (especially the peel, so use citrus zest for flavoring), carrots, cucumbers, peas, celery, and tomatoes. Pectin may prevent cancer cells from breaking away from the main tumor (metastasizing). While this would not eliminate a cancer, it could keep it from getting to other areas of our body, which is what makes a dangerous cancer deadly.

With pectin in so many fruits and vegetables, this may simply tell us that eating multiple servings of fruits and vegetables each day is good.

Other fiber-rich foods are leafy greens, which include lettuces, kale, spinach, collard greens, and chard, among others. These leafy greens are an excellent source of fiber, which is beneficial for the immune system. They are also high in carotenoids, which reduce oxidative damage in our body.

In addition to the fiber and carotenoids, leafy greens also contain folate and flavonoids, and are a good source of minerals, all of which are necessary for a healthy diet. Magnesium in particular is a mineral that is low in many of us. Magnesium is a cofactor for many enzymes, so low levels have many effects. Another source of minerals is in the water we drink. But many people now drink filtered and reverse osmosis (RO) water, so there is less mineral supply. Some ways to reverse this include salt baths (soaking in Epsom salts, for example) as well as eating more leafy greens or taking a mineral supplement that includes magnesium.

### Foods to Increase – Resveratrol

Resveratrol is a polyphenol that appears to give us beneficial action for reducing heart disease and cancer, likely due to its antioxidant action.

Red and purple grapes have a high level of resveratrol, as do dark berries, such as mulberries and blueberries. For this reason, these fruits, their juice, and red wines contain this compound. Because red wine includes fermentation with the grape skin, it has high levels of resveratrol. In addition to these fruits, cocoa powder (and dark chocolate) have high levels (second to red wine), with peanut skins and pistachio nuts next.

### Foods to Possibly Increase – Omega-3 Oils

There is evidence that omega-3 fatty acids, as found in the oils of many fish, help reduce the growth and spread of cancers. There is some concern about the source of the oils. One challenge with increasing consumption of fish is that many big fish also contain higher levels of mercury, which is toxic. Additionally, some farm-raised fish have been found to have polychlorinated biphenyls (PCBs) in their bodies, which is also toxic. The way to know if a fish has toxins is to use a guide like the one put out by the Monterey Bay Aquarium (Seafood Watch, available online and as a free app).

Other sources of omega-3 fatty acids include walnuts, flax oil, fish oil (cod liver oil, for example), and herbs and spices, such as marjoram, basil, oregano, tarragon, mint leaves, grape leaves, cloves, and capers, among others.

### Foods to Increase – Other Vegetables and Fruits

There are many other vegetables and fruits that are beneficial. The categories listed above are ones where we know how they work.

In general, eating fruits and vegetables is beneficial. Among the health advantages are compounds that protect us by removing free radicals with antioxidants, or improving cardiovascular function, or slowing the growth and spread of cancer, as with brightly colored berries and cruciferous vegetables. There are so many other health benefits from a wide variety of plants that a simple rule is to eat a variety of fruits and vegetables, have an abundance of these foods, and reduce our consumption of foods that are more harmful.

### Foods to Reduce

Not all foods are great, so let's look at ones we should reduce in our diet. These foods are ones that cause excessive inflammation. There is an updated listing of foods that have carcinogens on the American Cancer Society's site <http://www.cancer.org/Cancer/CancerCauses/OtherCarci nogens/GeneralInformationaboutCarcinogens/known-and-probable-human-carcinogens>. This gives much useful information about these compounds.

There are foods that are damaging to our bodies or that become damaging based on how we prepare them. These foods cause inflammation. Inflammation is our body's normal response to an injury. It makes the body mobilize white blood cells to fight infection and increases blood flow to that area. Inflammation also makes cells grow to help the healing. So inflammation is an important thing for healing in our body. When we eat burnt foods or processed foods with nitrates or nitrites, inflammation causes a large response in our body. This means we get more blood flow to that area and more cell growth. This all makes perfect sense when the irritant causing the inflammation is a cut – then we use this cell growth to repair the damage and heal. But when the damage is due to something that can cause a mutation of our cells, stimulating growth of these mutated cells can cause disease.

So while inflammation is a used to protect us from damage, it can also work against us when we have a potential mutagen in our body. You can picture it this way: If every day you wear shoes that have a small pebble under the right toe, you will gradually develop a callous in that spot. The irritation caused the skin to grow to protect the foot. But if this pebble were instead a mutagen, then this additional cell growth would make a mutation that is now in your body. This is how a good and normal process can cause problems.

Burnt foods are in this damaging category. Because of this, it is best to eliminate these from our diet, or at least to eat them rarely. Note that as with so many things that cause damage, eating less of it is important, and work toward not including it.

Other foods on this list to reduce or eliminate include many fried foods, particularly fried starches, such as potato chips or fries; alcohol, which is okay and can be beneficial when in small amounts (one or occasionally two glasses of red wine in a day) but is harmful in larger amounts; barbecue and burnt foods, which cause inflammation and contain carcinogens; and most meat. This latter one is difficult for many, as meat is a dietary staple for many of us.

The problem with meat is that it is high in fat, particularly saturated fat, and this causes our body to produce excess hormones, which can make cancers grow (particularly in the breast and prostate). Meat also lacks many of the protective compounds mentioned, such as fiber and other cancer-suppressing phytonutrients. Studies have shown that people with diets higher in meat have a greater risk of developing heart disease, high blood pressure, and cancers of the breast, prostate and colon (colon cancer is partly due to a lack of fiber, which slows the movement of food through the colon, exposing the colon to the irritants for a longer time).

As for fats, we need to eat omega-3 and omega-6 fats in similar amounts, since we need them for normal brain function and we cannot make them. But different foods have very different amounts of omega-6 to omega-3 fats. While fish generally have higher levels of omega-3 fats, land animals have higher levels of omega-6 fats. The amount changes based on what the animal ate. Choosing animals that were grass-fed rather than grain-fed will balance these fats. Grain-fed cattle have about 20:1 (omega-6:omega-3), and so do conventional eggs. Grass-fed cattle have a ratio of about 4:1, and eggs from range fed chickens are about 2:1. So while decreasing meat in your diet is best, it is good to choose grass-fed animals over grain-fed ones.

### Sun and Sleep and Stress

Two factors that play crucial roles in all this are rest and Vitamin D. Getting enough sleep each night helps our immune system respond well to stresses. When our immune system is working well, it is able to protect our body, so getting normal sleep each night and keeping to your normal pattern is good.

Just as rest is important for the immune system, so is Vitamin D. This is a compound we synthesize when our skin is exposed to the ultraviolet (UV) light of the sun. The part of the UV spectrum that is used for making Vitamin D is in the UVB range, around 300 nm. This allows our body to make Vitamin D, which then builds the immune system. Of course, too much sunlight can also be dangerous, as it can result in sunburns, which cause inflammation. So the best rule of thumb is to be in the sun much less time than it takes to burn. If your skin feels hotter afterward, you had too much exposure and need to decrease it in the future. So, Vitamin D is easy to add to our system – just go outside – but the minimum amount we need each day entails a modest time outside (fifteen minutes for many people).

When we have long-term stress in our life, this weakens our

immune system, upsets our digestive system, and dulls our thinking and memory. The reason is that our stress response releases the hormones adrenalin and cortisol into our body to get us energized to do things and these hormones shut down digestion and immune systems to be sure we have all energy available for action. Weakening digestion and immunity reduces our ability to digest our foods well and make it more likely we will get sick. These hormones decrease synapse creation, causing us to not make new memories.

It is wise to learn what can reduce your stress, and do it. Remember that what reduces stress for you this year may be different in another year, but always be aware of what you can do to reduce stress. Some common solutions include exercise of any type, prayer or meditation, sleep, reading or writing, drawing, painting, dancing or listening to music. Find what works for you and use it.

# Epilogue

We are all affected by chronic disease. We each will have close friends and family who will have cancer, heart disease, diabetes, and more. This book explains these conditions and our normal body function to provide benefit.

Second, anything we do can shift the odds for us to have healthier lives. We can increase our odds with regular activity, a healthy diet, regular medical checkups and immunizations, and by not smoking or vaping.

Third, activity is good for us. It boosts our immune system. Perhaps a good way to envision this is to remind yourself to get out and enjoy life: Spend time with friends, explore new and familiar places, keep active, and get good sleep every night. All of these help our immune system.

Fourth, our diet makes a difference. Eating foods that are high in antioxidants and other plant nutrients helps our body stay healthy. Reducing foods that stimulate inflammation is equally important. Opting for a healthy and moderate diet overall has lasting impact.

Finally, remember that what you do makes a difference, no matter when you start. It makes a difference in how you live life, and it will improve your odds for good health.

So, eat healthy, stay active and fit, avoid smoking, have fun, get rest, and enjoy your healthy and productive life.

# Index